WAVES
A DAY IN THE LIFE OF A SONOGRAPHER

WAVES

A Day in the Life of a Sonographer

CASSANDRA MCGINNITY

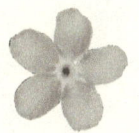

ISBN: 979-8-218-53285-7

Library of Congress Control Number: 2024921858

Dedicated to all the families who have lost a pregnancy, wished for a pregnancy, or were faced with an unimaginable struggle during those nine short months.

Fair warning: This story can be triggering for some individuals who may have experienced loss, infertility, or any other hardship during pregnancy and parenthood, but that being said, it can also be healing. Let's open up the conversation and allow each other the space to feel, support, and navigate through all of life's journeys.

Disclaimer: Although this is a memoir and based on real life events, the names and stories have been changed to protect the identities of patients and providers. This book is not intended as a substitute for the medical advice of physicians.

Introduction

THE FIRST time I had to tell someone their baby's heart had stopped, I almost quit. Within that same morning, I got the joyful pleasure of telling another couple that everything looked healthy with their baby boy. The intensity of that positive experience brought some sense of balance while I recovered from the whiplash of emotions. As a 24-year-old fresh out of college, my first day in the high-risk prenatal clinic felt grim and euphoric at the same time. It seems rather archaic to see life in only black and white, but thinking back, that's what a decade long career in ultrasound looks like. Exactly 256 shades of gray projected onto a monitor. Every single pixel and sound wave coming together to form an image that will determine the fate of so many lives.

Some people can only relate to ultrasound because of

pregnancy or seeing it on television, while others are familiar due to their own medical experience or backgrounds. Ultrasound is like a Trojan horse. It is disguised in the media as babies, gender reveals, and happy stories, but in reality it is also cancer diagnoses and fetal demises. From a morning of happy tears and elation to an afternoon of heartache and devastation. My patients need someone. Someone to celebrate with, someone to cry with; simply someone to give their all during part of life's most extreme moments. Regardless of the constant ups and downs and emotional stress, I am forever grateful that I get to be that someone.

Throughout this story I will reflect on one day in the ultrasound unit of the high risk prenatal office. If you can imagine multiplying this day by about 250 per year for ten years, that is the pressure and significance I want to exhibit. Although one day cannot, by any means, encompass all the encounters in the prenatal ultrasound world, it can give insight: enough to humble the ignorant, teach things to those who want more knowledge, bring awareness to the ultrasound career, relatability to those who have had similar stories, and honor the love and loss that surrounds every single patient story.

WAVES
A DAY IN THE LIFE OF A SONOGRAPHER

7:08 a.m.

I ALWAYS show up to work in a fluster. Three bags hanging off my arms, a coffee borderline spilling in one hand and an ID badge that is at the bottom of my never-ending purse. Rummaging through my bag to find the key to the door is my first stressor of the day, which is totally within my control, but I choose to throw it in the depths of the large sack every single night after work. My day starts and ends with punching the time clock since I am an hourly employee; thank God for that. If I didn't have the physical and metaphorical luxury of being "on" and "off" the clock I don't think I would have lasted this long in the medical field.

Once inside and clocked in for the day I can navigate my way to my ultrasound room, throw my belongings into the cupboard under the sink and start my day. I log onto my computer, and about twelve other software programs within, okay maybe only three but I swear it feels like more when I am already stressed and I haven't even seen patients yet today. The bright lights of the screen make my eyes retract in disgust. Being a sonographer means I work better in the dark, ironically I always say to my patients, "Let me turn the lights down so that I can see." This might be one of the only careers that this funny fact applies to.

There have already been two staff call outs today so I know it is going to be a hellacious day. We usually run with a skeleton crew anyway, never mind with employees calling out. That basically means there will be no time to breathe, drink water, or eat lunch for my nine hour shift. Perfect, just like every other day around here. I am not sure if I have always been this sarcastic or if working in the medical field forty plus hours a week has morphed me into some *Chandler Bing* wannabe.

I make sure my room is stocked with as many basic white cotton towels as I can shove into the broken, half-painted drawers and as much ultrasound gel as I can physically fit into the designated plastic containers that are for "liquid" items only. I will not go into infection control protocols as that is a whole different beast to discuss. Between the constant site visits from staffers in a button down shirt or skirts and heels and the chaotic mess that is clean versus dirty utility rooms, there is just too much to dissect.

Just like with construction plans, no one ever asks the employees who actually work in the trenches each and every day. Someone in a sterile room with a hot coffee and sun shining through their spacious office window is making decisions about things that they have little to no idea about, other than didactic logistical knowledge. I swear every career should have didactics and some sort of hands-on-training. Every damn career, not just those that are medically oriented. Not that it will help much, but it would be a step in the right direction if you ask me.

Finally, I turn on my ultrasound machine and the patient viewing monitor attached to the wall before assessing the extent of my schedule for the day. The office where I work runs about 13 ultrasound rooms each day, which means 13 sonographers are needed to staff every one of those rooms daily. I rotate locations between an IVF clinic, the hospital, the outpatient facility, and another offsite. Today, I am at the outpatient facility, but it also isn't unheard of for me to be expected in two places at once.

The outpatient office has seven of those ultrasound rooms. Today I am assigned to be in room three of seven. I open up my assigned schedule after taking two longer than average sips of my coffee. I close my eyes and angle my gaze towards the ceiling as an internal affirmation that I got this and I can get through this day. Then, I open my eyes and begin the chaos.

As I sit in this less than ergonomically correct chair, I can feel the rage start to bubble up as soon as I see the massive amount of exams that are scheduled in my room. Let me put it into perspective: a busy day doesn't necessarily consist of the number of patients, but the reasons why each patient is being seen, which is termed the "indication of exam." My schedule today is peppered with over-booked appointments and possible fetal abnormalities seen at outside facilities, which means I will definitely need to be in two places at once. I take a deep breath, refocus on my inner mantras, and click on the first patient chart of the day.

This particular patient is here for a routine fetal survey exam. The American College of Obstetricians and Gynecologists recommends that every pregnant patient receive an 18-22 week anatomy scan to rule out any fetal anomalies. This scan tells the doctors that there is no severe structural abnormality that could impact the quality of life for the fetus outside of the womb. Yes, I know this scan is usually known, in the non-medical world, as the "gender scan" or the "appointment where you find out if it is a boy or girl," but let me tell you, it is *so* much more than that. Let me repeat this fact: *it is so much more than that.* If I can get anything out into the world it would be the mere fact that this scan is not, I repeat not, the "gender scan." This scan, in some instances, determines the immediate fate of that tiny human growing inside its mother's womb. This scan is so important and has made an incredible difference in the world of fetal science and maternal mortality rates. If you decide to only get one ultrasound during your entire pregnancy I suggest this one. Not that I am a qualified practitioner that can recommend this, so this is not medical advice, just friendly sonographer advice.

I click through about fourteen screens before actually being able to see the information that is necessary to start the scan on the computer. Why oh why technology. We love it and we hate it, although I guess I really wouldn't have a job without it.

I finally get to the patient chart and of course the information that I need is not provided by the referring doctor, nor did they bother to put an order in. Perfect, let me just do your work for you, another aspect of the medical field that leaves a sour taste in my mouth. Sure, it may be way more multifactorial than that but still I allow myself this little outburst of opinions. Maybe it's just the big corporation hospitals that are so large they cannot organize all the small details, but it still makes things very frustrating for us down here on the front lines. Again, an instance where asking the people who are actually doing the work might bring enormous benefits to both parties, but alas this common sense is not yet enforced. *Sigh.*

When I can finally leave my room to walk down the hallway towards the waiting room it is about ten minutes later than the patient's appointment time. This is a common occurrence, which leaves both me and the patient in a frustrated state even before we meet each other. I swear the mental strength it takes to get through the day in the medical field is herculean. Do this, do that, don't do this, but do that even though we just told you not to, pretty much sums up what every day consists of from management.

I walk down the hallway, lined with doors and wall hand sanitizers placed strategically every two feet, towards the waiting room. Every time I walk down this hallway I find myself reflecting in an almost sarcastic tone about the devastation and joy that takes place in each of these rooms. Without the ability to let go or block things out, none of us would make it a week in medicine. It just wouldn't work. How are you supposed to go from telling someone their lives will forever be changed to then immediately go home to your healthy happy family? You can't, unless you can place it in a compartment or sarcastic sentence that you can pretend isn't real.

As I walk down the hallway I pass by one of the physicians. I always find energy through the contempt to say hello or good morning, but they never fail to continue to walk by without a hint of eye contact. My eyes speak for us both as they roll in the back of my head after they pass me. Yes, my eyes get tired from the amount of eye rolling I do in a day, thank you for being concerned. I probably walk about six to eight miles a day down these hallways. You read that right: six to eight miles and my Apple watch doesn't lie, as far as I know. Patients always make the comment "this place is a maze" even though we literally walk down one "L" shaped hallway from the waiting room to the exam room. It is a long hall, don't get me wrong, but in no way a corn field.

As I open the waiting room door to call for my patient my mind is in five different places. I try to remember if I forgot to turn the coffee pot off this morning, half of my lunch is still on the kitchen counter, damn, and I forgot to put my badge on. Oops. Also slightly an oxymoron isn't it? I remember that I forgot, I always thought that was an interesting play on words.

Opening the door to the waiting room always signals a sort of either fear or bliss of the unknown. What is behind that door? A full waiting room? No one? A couple people? One person? A monster, who knows?

Waiting rooms in any area of the medical field serve pretty much the same purpose. Whether it is in the emergency department or at the local physician's office, waiting rooms all serve as a placeholder. A room for patients that is convenient, decently comfortable, and reasonably clean. The walls are usually bare or have minimal decorations. The tables are not only lined with germs, but medical pamphlets that seem overly tenacious. Hand sanitizer is readily available on every surface and the chairs are sectioned out strategically, allowing for maximum capacity in the given space.

The problem with waiting rooms is that humans are nosy and needy. It is in our nature to be curious and inquisitive, so things like HIPAA (Health Insurance Portability and Accountability Act) exist to protect the most private details from one person to another. There are signs and posters to gently ask each individual to wait behind the line for the receptionist to call them forward, yet there still seems to be at least one person who fails to read it. This creates a fascinating environment where one person is anxiously waiting to be called next due to being late for work and another patient is anxiously waiting to be called because she is finding out her results from her biopsy. These are the details that HIPAA protects, so the emotions may be similar but the reason is on a totally different spectrum from patient to patient.

The waiting room door resembles more than just an entrance to the scheduled appointment. It represents a barrier from the outside world to the world of decisions, trauma, excitement, disappointment, and expectations. The symbolism of that door means more than the physical legality of the obstruction. Compartments within our brains and within our lives are sometimes the key to maintaining emotional and physical homeostasis. These compartments can be an object, such as a door, that is easily seen, or an internal switch that is regulated by only one's self. At times these barriers fall and we as humans are what we consider to be vulnerable. To be vulnerable is to let someone else hold the key to one of our own compartments. Humans do this on a daily basis both consciously and subconsciously. The simple act of walking into the patient entrance through the waiting room door is theoretically the same idea as handing over a key to a part of one's self to the medical professional. The patient is subconsciously saying, "Here is the key to my future child, please use it carefully, skillfully, and compassionately." Without saying those exact words or even truly knowing it, this is what each patient who walks into an ultrasound appointment is doing.

The trouble with this is that every patient who hands over the key to their growing fetus is not the same by any means. The emotional diversity of the women's health and prenatal population is so vast, it expands far beyond the barriers of one single compartment. This leads to a situation of organized chaos during the nine short months of pregnancy. A patient hands over one key but several keys are needed to adequately understand and care for each individual patient. During a time of unexpected life-threatening news it's almost as if there was no key ever made to access a compartment for this kind of despair. The sonographer performing the ultrasound quickly shuffles through his or her own keychain for answers that can not be found.

The waiting room at the maternal fetal medicine office is unlike any other. It houses women who are visually pregnant, women who are struggling to conceive, and women of all ages there for routine appointments. Some days I try to embody how the women who are having trouble trying to conceive feel when they are sitting in a waiting room full of pregnant women. Does it bother them at all? Does it make them feel sad, uneasy, happy, hopeful? Do not underestimate waiting rooms. This is the first mistake I ever made. When patients are waiting for their name to be called it's as if they will answer to any name. I could call "Ashley" from the waiting room door and a random patient would stand up and ask, "Did you say Megan?"

I look at the clock on the far wall as I swing open the door to the waiting room; 7:08 a.m., late already. I call for my first patient of the day.

"Jessica," I say. Jessica and her partner stand up, looking eager, both with smiles on their faces.

I look around to make sure three other people don't rise out of their seats with her. Jessica is a fairly common name after all.

As I lead them down the hallway to our ultrasound room, she asks to use the restroom. I point to a door to our left and continue down the hallway towards our room, her husband still trailing behind me.

The hallway leading to each ultrasound room is long and narrow with all the rooms in one corridor. These seven ultrasound rooms house patients of all different gestational ages, numbers, and situations. Each room has a different story, different family, and different emotions. We turn into ultrasound room three and I direct Jessica's husband to the chair next to the exam table. Brief moments with the patient's partners are always interesting. Some like to discuss the weather, while others make it known to me the wishes of their partner before she even enters the room. I am uncertain if this is out of nervousness or genuine care, however some are more adamant than others. I usually just nod and reiterate my same questions to the patient when she returns. I can hear Jessica flush the toilet followed by the shuffling of her feet down the hall. *Thank God*, I think to myself, the awkward silence or minimal conversation with the partner is never short enough.

In the medical field it is rare to find a patient that doesn't have questions, but Jessica and her husband seem content for the time being. I confirm her date of birth and last name and ask her to lie down on the exam table.

For some reason the patient always comes to the left side of the table to sit down, the side where I sit and my ultrasound machine is parked. Why is it so difficult for a patient to get on the table from the right side? Is it out of muscle memory or is it an actual physical limitation? This has clearly happened enough to cause some annoyance.

Anyway, Jessica slowly lays back, not without a few grunts and breath holds. I can see the grimace on her face when she finally makes it into a somewhat adequate position.

Good enough, is the face she's making, however due to the ergonomical demands of ultrasound I ask, "Could you please just scoot over on the table towards me a bit more?"

Jessica does scoot, as they all do, thankfully, but I always do feel slightly awful for asking this. Then I think about my daily shoulder pain and the long road I still have in my career. I convince myself that having a patient scoot a couple inches to the right is nothing comparatively. I usually end up scanning between ten to sixteen patients a day. I was unaware of the physical demands of this career until I was in too deep.

I remember the instructors in school constantly telling us to watch our ergonomics and I would always brush it off like it was nonsense. Well, two employee health stents and a boat load of chiropractic bills later I can say it is not nonsense. The ultrasound career has taken away my ability to sleep on my right side, go bowling, and some nights use my right hand to brush my teeth. But, however painful, I wake up the next day and show up to work again.

Jessica and her husband seem truly excited about the ultrasound. This is their first pregnancy and they just informed me they have been trying to conceive for over a year now. So, yes, an extremely exciting and happy time for these two parents to be. I can see the positive emotions beaming from both of their faces as Jessica looks over at her husband and they hold hands, waiting eagerly for the first glimpses of their baby.

There is a patient viewing screen mounted on the wall in front of the exam table. This is such an important tool for the patients to be able to comfortably see the exam as I am scanning. Before this glorious invention the patients would ask constantly to see my screen while I was scanning, which is borderline impossible. I would have a broken neck and a bum shoulder by lunch time. However convenient this extra screen is, it can also be quite tragic if for some reason there is something noticeably wrong, even by the layman's eye. Humans can sense when something is wrong even if words are not exchanged. I do my best to stay stoic until I know the actuality of the situation, but that is not always the easiest.

Jessica's husband seems quite nervous; I can see him sitting on the edge of his chair with his fingers now clasped together. I am sure he is equally excited, but the emotions, nonetheless, are palpable.

As I subtly witness the joy in both of their faces I slowly put on my two gloves to begin the exam. I hand Jessica two bleach white towels and ask her to tuck one into her waist band down low and one under her shirt up high. It never fails, women are always self conscious, even if they *literally* look like supermodels. I swear they tuck the towels in and leave me about one inch of skin to scan on, at about the level of the belly button. This is your first lesson in uterine anatomy. The uterus is not in your chest, it is down low in your pelvis. Like *really* low, in between your hip bones. Not under the belly button, not under the breast bones, low like the low rise jeans I wore in the 2000's low.

"Could you please pull your pants down a little lower off your hips?" I ask.

Jessica tugs and groans, but manages to get her pant line far enough down so that my transducer can get an accurate image. I grab the bottle of gel that is now set on the side of my machine in a little warming canister, how fancy. This is a fairly new but not groundbreaking feature of the ultrasound machines. Of course it depends what model you have, and let me tell you they can be ancient, but being in maternal fetal medicine has its perks and we usually get the best of the best as far as technology goes.

As I am squirting the gel on her belly her husband squeals.

"Is it cold?" he asks.

I hear this question at least ten times a day. He asks it in a sort of laughing school girl undertone, which is just hilarious. Men, if they only knew what it felt like as women to go through what we go through, but you can't blame them too much as they literally just have no idea. Finally, I grab my probe and settle into the most ergonomic friendly position that I can initially.

Jessica is 20 weeks along, which means I should be able to see most of the baby with ease. When the image first shows up, everyone is always expecting to see the quintessential photo of a fetus; the cute profile picture, or the baby sucking on its thumb or toes. However, this is far from the actuality of the scan. The first things I look for are any major abnormalities, number of babies and the presence or absence of a heartbeat. I have learned my lesson and now, before anything else, I always show the patient the heart beat first before obtaining any other images. This at least settles most patients for the time being.

As I skillfully place the probe down on Jessica's stomach I see the heart beating, *thank God*; 134 beats per minute, very normal.

Not even a second after I start scanning I hear Jessica ask, "Does everything look normal?"

I wish I could tell if everything looked normal in one second. That would save my arm a hell of a lot of pain and my brain a whole lot of stress. Unfortunately, in order to determine if things are looking normal it takes about 45 minutes, sometimes longer depending if the fetus would like to cooperate or not.

"We will be looking at all the different parts of the baby today and going over them together, you will have a better idea of it all at the end of the appointment," I say with a smile.

After I explain this to her I start to examine what I like to call the "non-baby parts" first. I like to get the lay of the land, so to speak, before assessing the entire fetus head to toe. First I check her cervix, then the placenta and her ovaries. I quickly scan through the uterus to check the fluid level and finally get started on the anatomy of the baby.

"Would you like to know the sex of the baby today?" I ask Jessica and her husband, taking a second to quickly glance in their direction.

They both look at each other for about five seconds with matching unsure smiles, but ultimately agree.

"Yes," they say in unison.

Sometimes the fetus will show me what I need to see right away and other times it may take awhile. If the baby gives the genitalia up right away I will take the picture as quickly as possible, because if I miss my chance that's going to be one upset mama and I don't have time for that today. Even though I might take the "gender" picture first, I still need to make sure this squirmy bag of bones and organs is normal before revealing the exciting news. In order to get the right view to see the sex, the fetus must open its legs, yes, literally, and let me see between. It either has a penis or it doesn't, however you'll be surprised by the amount of times I have told patients they were having the latter when they were told from another facility it was a boy/girl. That is one surprise that is never fun.

This could happen due to the scan being performed too early in gestational age, the fetus not cooperating, or just sonographer error; either way the unexpected in the prenatal world is not usually fun. The entirety of this exam is so important, literally every single detail. Down to even the tiny finger bones. I think I scan through things fifteen times before I actually take the picture or call it normal. Because that's the nature of this job, if we don't see it then the doctor doesn't see it, and to be totally honest ultrasound can fool you, especially since we are scanning live and only the still images go to the doctors. Almost daily I look back at an image that I took only a few hours prior and could still get confused. This is why we go to school for so long and why real time scanning is so crucial.

We are about 15 minutes into the exam. So far everything is looking good; if there were a major abnormality I would have seen a glimpse of it by now. The baby has shown me its spine, its fingers and toes, its brain and a basic view of its heart. Good enough for now. I usually let the patient know how everything looks after each part is evaluated, that way their nerves can be calmed ever so slightly as we continue the exam. That's another thing about maternal fetal medicine ultrasound, we are allowed and encouraged to tell patients results, both normal and abnormal. It is part of our jobs as sonographers; we work extremely close with the doctors and they trust us. This is also why the training is so much more intense.

Finally the baby shows me in between its legs. It's a boy. It is always a sort of weird but special feeling knowing this little bit of knowledge even before the parents do. Like who am I to be able to have this information? Pretty cool, and I do not take that for granted. I take a deep breath and look over at the two parents. Their mouths are open and they are baiting my every breath.

"It's a boy!" I tell them with fake but also genuine excitement.

It's true I am genuinely happy for them, but also I do this ten times a day, so the fairytale wears off with time. I have to keep my emotions in check, one slip up and I'll either be crying with my patient or getting an invite to their gender reveal party, both of which would be highly inappropriate on a professional level, however flattering.

The best part of my job is when the ultrasound is normal. Normal is good, normal is easy, normal means I go home on time. Everyone wants normal. In the ultrasound hall of this office, at any given time, there could be seven rooms all with positive news or seven rooms with the latter. Usually it is a mix between them both, truly it could be a 50/50 situation, seeing as this is the high risk ward of pregnancy. If the mother or fetus is high risk in any way, this is where you would be seen for your prenatal care, at least in this state, as there is only one within the entire region, so we are it for you, you don't have a choice, sorry. I mean we are the best of the best let's be honest, but if you were a patient in let's say, Boston, Massachusetts, you would have multiple options of maternal fetal care instead of just one.

I finish up the exam looking at the arms, legs and other internal organs.

"The spine is looking great, the brain looks wonderful and this little guy has a normal heart. His legs and arms just barely slowed down enough for me to catch them, but everything is looking great," I say.

I show the parents the baby's nose and lips and the profile picture, and they both beam and try to envision the three dimensional version of the little cherub. Discussing who's nose and ears it has and joking about the possibilities of hair color. Again, normal is easy.

It never fails, usually when I show the profile picture the parents ask, "Well, can we see the face?" As if I can go in there and whip out an HD picture of exactly what the fetus looks like. I swear some patients expect the image to look borderline cartoonish. When I have a perfectly normal profile picture on the screen and they are still asking me if they can see the face, what are they expecting? An emoji-like image? A real life photography image? I am never quite sure. I usually just keep scanning in hopes they move on to something else.

Thankfully Jessica and her husband have most likely seen ultrasound pictures before and accept the cute profile picture with wide smiles that fill the room with pure joy.

Everything is looking within normal limits. I let out a brief breath of relief and check the time. 7:52 a.m., perfect timing. Rarely do I say that, but thank God because I know how the rest of my day is predicted to go based on my quick peek at the schedule this morning. I place the probe back on the ultrasound machine and let Jessica clean off the excess gel that is on her stomach.

The comment "Good thing I am going home to shower after this" is a very common response at the end of the exam and Jessica follows suit. Dang, if I felt that dirty after just a little bit of sterile gel on my skin, I would be showering like 12 times a day, probably more. Maybe they should install one here for patients to use after their ultrasounds? For me to hide out and sleep in? No? A girl can dream.

Jessica swings her legs over the side of the bed, kisses her husband and they both smile and thank me multiple times.

"Thank you so much, we are thrilled," Jessica says as she is grabbing her things.

Sometimes patients even give me a hug at the end of this exam when they are just so relieved that everything is okay. This single handedly makes my day, like nothing else at my job, I am all for hugs and human connection. The pure gratefulness of my expertise and honest happiness that everything is normal makes it all worth it. I find it hard to use that word anymore, "normal," other than in the medical field. Here we use that word daily, and it is the only word you want to hear when you are inside the walls of hospitals. But in the rest of the world it seems that word is fading in its definition, for better or worse.

Other times after exams, patients leave angry because the sex of the baby is not what they predicted. Really? The odds are 50/50 for every human on the planet that can conceive naturally. This makes my blood boil. Seeing parents or one parent visibly showing signs of disgust towards their unborn child, for something they themselves created, full well knowing their odds, is just down right gross. And when I say visibly showing, I truly mean it. From a dad who has been chatty the whole ultrasound to completely shutting down or the mom who is actually crying because it's a boy and not a girl. Listen, I understand wanting something and not getting it, but this is a human being we are talking about here, not a new pair of shoes. Gender disappointment is real, and it's okay to be upset, feel your feelings, etc.; but it's not okay to treat me or others with disrespect/Isn't this what they teach toddlers? What happened, you didn't get your way and now you're reverting back?

I hand the printed ultrasound pictures to Jessica and walk towards the exit to show them out.

"Take care, it was so nice to meet you," I say as I show them out the door and into the hallway.

I am known to give way too many ultrasound pictures, I mean way too many, according to my managers, but the patients can never have enough. The exam room door opens directly into the ultrasound wing. I am leading Jessica and her husband down the hall when I look up and see the bright blue water teardrop sign taped on the outside of the door of ultrasound room six. My heart instantly drops. The only thing that sign indicates is sad, abnormal, awful news. A first time parent with normal news wouldn't know this, but I know this and my insides curl up and ache for the news that is being delivered only 20 feet away. Again through a door, actual or metaphorical it doesn't matter; I know what tragic information is being discussed.

I take a quick breath in and out to clear my immediate thoughts and continue to show Jessica down the hallway towards the exit. As we walk the hall we pass another couple who is walking in the other direction, tears in their eyes. For a moment I make eye contact with the woman. Her eyelids are heavy, her lips drawn down, and she has a tissue in one of her hands. She is hurrying along and seemingly trying to leave as quickly as she can, her partner trailing behind. She looks at me in a way that says, this is the worst day of my life thus far. It is almost like a slow-motion part of a movie, where her eyes slowly meet mine and then slowly shift back toward the floor in front of her.

I am unsure if my patient and her partner were aware of the two situations simultaneously taking place as we exited our room that was filled with calmness and joy, but I am. I am always aware.

I keep walking, gently point to the exit door and genuinely smile from deep down in my gut as I say a final farewell to this lovely couple. They may or may not know just how lucky they are. It is far too real for me, as are the daily ups and downs here, and possibly far too surreal for them. Either way, this is a harsh reality of prenatal ultrasound, especially in the high-risk division. Not every couple leaves this office with a smile on their faces. Actually, a good percentage of people leave with worry, devastation, or fear. A healthy baby and a healthy mama is the goal of every provider in this practice, but that is not always what the universe has in store, unfortunately.

8:01 a.m.

BY THE time I get back to my room, clean and disinfect it for the next patient, it is already past the next appointment time. Shocker, didn't I already predict this would be the case all day? I reach over the counter to grab another cloth to finish cleaning. The disinfecting wipes that we use have time limits, two minutes for that surface, ten minutes for this one. I have to wait the allotted time after wiping anything clean in order for the table and surfaces to dry. It gets confusing keeping up with all the numbers, so I usually just call it an even ten minutes before I can grab my next patient. Not that the scheduling powers that be take any of this extra time into account. I look back at the schedule on my computer screen. My eyes already hurt and my brain is in too many different places at once to focus. Through my blurry vision, I see the next patient is here for a routine third-trimester position check. Thank God, I think to myself, this is as easy as it can get. I was already ten minutes late and I didn't need another long exam to follow my first. My arm is already tired.

I think back for a moment to the woman who just walked through the halls, teary-eyed, and picture the sadness that lurks behind the door in room six. I sort of zone out for a second in front of my computer screen. The lights from the monitor are bright so I stare down towards the floor in front of me. No matter how long you work in prenatal women's health, the sadness you see on these women's faces when something is wrong just stays with you for longer than anyone would like. As the saying goes, try not to bring work home with you, but how are we supposed to do that when literally you are changing the outcome of someone's life in mere minutes?

I snap out of it and glance back at the exam table I just cleaned to make sure it has dried enough to pull the table paper down for the next patient. Usually once per day, each one of us will see something that is just heart wrenching, whether it's a change in birth plan or a change in life plan. There are no words that best describe the emotions and the energy during those changes because it is so vastly different from person to person and case to case.

In school the teachers would teach us some of the rare

abnormalities that we could encounter in our careers. Each time they would say, "Oh, but you will never see this, it's super rare." Thinking back, I have seen almost every single rare thing that I was ever taught. At first, I thought there is no way that I will see any of this, but when you work in the only high risk prenatal center in the state for nearly ten years, you see a lot and a little of everything. I have seen everything from conjoined twins to natural quintuplets. Talk about one in a million, try one in sixty million.

My room is in somewhat decent order so I swiftly make my way back down the hallway towards the waiting room. Every time I walk down this hallway I slip into a not so surreal reality. Memories of moments spent in each of these rooms, good, bad, and uncertain. I glance from room two to room five to four, knowing full well what happens behind these doors. We change lives, for the better and for the worse. The information we deliver is life changing. Sometimes I am surprising a patient with the news of twins and other times I am solemnly telling parents there is no heartbeat in the mere weeks before they were set to deliver.

I make a slight shaking motion of my head to remove these memories once again and briefly close my eyes to erase the thoughts compounding in my brain as I stand outside the waiting room door. My brain needs a clean slate before I start a new patient exam; at least emotionally. I push open the door and take a quick glance at the clock, late again, but this should be fast, so I tell myself.

My next patient is ready and waiting for me. I pause. I just need one more second, mainly to remember her name before calling for her. She is a young woman who is in the final weeks of her third trimester. She has one healthy child already and this will be her second. I swear I do too much chart reading and digging. God, I wish all the pertinent information I need would be easy to access, but apparently that's not how these electronic medical charts are developed, or perhaps it's user error; I'll just leave that statement right there for you to decide.

Her referring physician scheduled an ultrasound to check the position of the baby. In the third trimester, in order to be cleared for a vaginal birth, the fetus needs to be head down in the pelvis. This fetal presentation is termed "cephalic" or "vertex" in medical terminology. This is a pretty well known fact among pregnant women and this specific ultrasound indication is common in the third trimester. If the fetus is bottom down, this is termed "breech" presentation, and the physician will usually recommend a c-section. I am not a physician by a long shot, but I do know that non-head down deliveries are extremely rare in this day and age. Not impossible, as midwives and other advanced practice professionals are performing them, however just not as common. There are lots of opinions on this, as there are in lots of areas of medicine, so seeing as I do not have an "MD" at the end of my name I will only refer to the knowledge that I have gleaned for recommendations from physicians working in the field of maternal fetal medicine.

"Anna," I say loud enough so everyone can hear me.

Anna stands up from her chair with both hands supporting the weight of her and her unborn child on the arm rests. Her face grimacing as she stands, her husband gently helping her to her feet. She waddles over to me with a tired smile on her face. I hold the door for them as they walk past me into the back of the office. In the third trimester, understandably, women are usually walking slightly slower at this point. So, I casually pretend to walk slower as I small talk with the couple before arriving at our ultrasound room.

"Did you all drive far to get here today?" I ask.

"Not too bad, only about 30 minutes," Anna replies.

Anna is 38 weeks pregnant. She is basically full term and I am sure she is ready to have this baby any day now. The exhaustion in the end is so intense, from insomnia to the constant wondering as to when the little bundle of joy will make their grand entrance. Every little hiccup or backache makes you question, *is this it, is this labor?* Especially if it's your first child.

The unknown of pregnancy and labor is something that is not talked about enough. Women and couples have so many opinions, but truth be told every pregnancy and every delivery is different. Every single one. Yes, even if there are millions of births a day, they are still all extremely different. Which is the way it should be to be honest; everyone has their own experience and their own hopes and dreams in this world, why would the birth of a new human be any different?

Pregnancy and child birth is your narrative, no one else's, live this story exactly as you want, utilize the village and accept help from others but stay true to yourself and you will never be wrong.

From the mom who has a birth plan that has been written in stone since the day she peed on a stick to the mom who goes into the hospital with zero expectations and almost delivers in the elevator on the way to the delivery room, the reality is this: delivering a child, as normal as it may seem, is anything but. The experience, the feelings, the changes, all of it factor in to make one big memory. Your memory, my memory, no one else's. So, as much as I agree that pregnancy and a woman's body should be discussed and educated about more, I also think it is so tough to try to relate differing birth stories to gain more control over the unknown. A birth story will always be untold until it happens.

We enter the room and I head towards my computer to start the basic necessities of the patient's care. Name, date of birth, etc., etc. Anna lets out a big sigh as she throws her purse over the back of the guest chair and slumps down onto the exam table. I glance over at her as I finish up asking her the pertinent questions.

She looks up at me and says, "Please tell me this child is head down and I will go into labor tonight."

Her husband clicks his tongue and takes a seat in the designated chair beside Anna.

"She has been doing everything to jump start it, you name it and she has done it. I even have packets of hot sauce in my pockets right now," he says chuckling. I laugh.

"We are going to check the position of the baby today, and make sure everything else looks good," I say to her, hoping to ease some of her anxiety.

Her husband looks like he is either going to pass out from fear or fall asleep at this point. His head is bobbing up and down and his eyelids look heavy. I quietly try to ignore that situation, seeing as he is safely seated in a chair, and start my ultrasound.

Anna is lying down and ready to start. I apply some

ultrasound gel on her belly and begin the exam.

As I said before, the first picture that I always take is the heart rate, so I quickly get that; 132 beats per minutes, normal. I move the probe inferior near Anna's lower belly. My eyes glued to my screen and my right hand in an almost death grip on the probe. I swear I need to work on my ergonomics more or my career is going to be over in no time. As I focus on the image on my screen I see that the baby is in fact breech. I see the bladder and the bum down low in Anna'a pelvis. The black and white screen can determine so much in so little time. I have literally only taken two pictures and these results are going to disappoint Anna.

The couple is waiting very patiently for my first words. I turn slightly towards Anna and her husband;

"Your baby is breech," I say with some hesitance.

Anna doesn't speak right away, but then her husband asks, "So, what does that mean?"

Anna replies with a short tone, "It means I have to have a c-section Adam, that's what it means."

She is disappointed and he is oblivious.

At this point, I can pretty much deduce that this is a huge change to Anna's birth plan. Whether this information comes from a controlled situation, as in right now or in the form of an emergency unexpected c-section, it is a change and Anna was not prepared for it.*

Yes, there are things like external cephalic version and spinning babies; however these may or may not work. There are also some midwives who are trained enough, and know enough to deliver babies breech, if the conditions are optimal as I stated previously, but this option is not always safe for everyone. IF, being the key word here. I am all for keeping birth plans and avoiding c-sections. The National Health Institutes published an article in May 2023 detailing the fact that too many are being done in this country unnecessarily right now anyway. But, the goal is to keep mom and baby safe. Period. This includes preventing a major surgery that may not be needed or having a major surgery because it is in fact very much needed.

In Anna's case she is very close to the end of her pregnancy, most likely her doctor will recommend c-section as the safest delivery option, given her amniotic fluid levels are also on the subjectively low side. So, yes in this case, major surgery will most likely be the safest option for both mom and baby, which is again always number one. Without adequate fluid levels surrounding the baby, this puts the fetus at higher risk

---

* After becoming a mother myself, the one thing I have learned over all else is that when it comes to pregnancy and birth, sometimes we do not have as much control as we think we have.

for a poor outcome.

I glance over quickly to look at Anna's face. I am having a hard time reading between the frown lines and pursed lips, but my gut feeling is that this news might be the worst thing to happen to her during this pregnancy. Of course, in my brain I think this is the least of her worries, but Anna hasn't been exposed to all the harsh realities that can happen during pregnancy like I have, thank God for that.*

I let the news settle in with Anna and Adam for a beat and turn to continue my exam, my eyes now solely focused on the fetus and uterus on my screen. I move my hand holding the transducer to the top of Anna's belly and can see the round shape of the baby's skull. *Oh, that must be so uncomfortable,* I think to myself. I can physically feel the hard, round area underneath my probe. Ouch.

Anna turns towards me and asks, "Can I get some pictures of the face?"

This is my least favorite question. Okay, I know what you all are thinking, why is this my least favorite question?

---

* During my own pregnancy I was so sick every day that I did not have the energy or time to think too much about everything. All I could think about was where I was going to vomit next. When I think back on this, it was probably in my favor, because if I was constantly questioning and thinking about everything I know too much about, I would have made myself crazy. I think my sickness really made me ignore everything I knew too much about during pregnancy. A blessing in disguise if you ask me.

Not because I don't want to provide the couple with a cute picture to take home, but because nine times out of ten it is impossible to get the picture they are expecting me to get. This could be due to the baby's position, maternal body habitus, or low amniotic fluid levels. Under optimal conditions at this late gestational age it is hard to see the face. Nevermind for someone like Anna who has a breech baby with minimal fluid. More than likely a picture is not going to happen today, at least not the picture they envision.

I can usually grab a picture of the feet or a close up of the nose and lips or hand, but rarely the quintessential profile picture at this stage in the game. It is basically impossible to capture anything that is visible to the non-ultrasound eye. I would love to get the perfect 2D and 3D picture of the baby's face for every couple that I encounter, but unfortunately that is not the case in the least. These reasons are precisely why I dislike the question. If the baby is in the perfect position with the perfect amount of fluid in front of its face, it is like a dream come true and I am thrilled to give multiple pictures to the parents.

After Anna asks, I try my hardest to get a picture but alas, all the fetus wants to do is look straight down towards Anna's spine and not budge. Patients will do almost anything to get that first glimpse of the baby and Anna is no exception. She tries to roll around and do a couple of jumping jacks, but still the baby does not want to show us their face. I set the probe down on the machine and I can almost hear Anna sigh in annoyance either at the fact that the baby is breech or that I could not capture the Instagram worthy picture for her; likely both. Her husband seems to have startled in the chair next to her, as if just waking up from a mid winter's nap.

Not only is Anna's baby breech but her fluid levels measured low, which means I must go review this scan with the reading physician.

"I'll be right back, I just need to go review this with the doctor," I say to the couple before walking out of the room to track down a physician, which is no easy task.

On any given day, we could have one to four physicians in the office, however each of them are assigned different duties. Let me just tell you when I say, if the physician you find isn't the one reading ultrasound today, then they will not be helping you in your time of need, period. I mean, I get it, we are all busy but holy moly sometimes these patients wait upwards of 45 minutes for me to beg one of the alternate doctors to review the scan. This puts my schedule massively behind and the next patient ends up in the waiting room for extended minutes, or even hours, past their exam time. Now, there is a caveat to this logistical nightmare of a process. In the prenatal world we work fast, and this is precisely because there are only nine short months of pregnancy, so waiting for results doesn't really cut it in this neck of the woods. In general ultrasound, you could get a scan of your liver and may not get results from a doctor for upwards of two weeks. We can't do that here, clearly. If this baby or mama is in distress we are working hard and fast to make sure they are safe right now, not in two weeks. That being said, even when patients do have to wait upwards of 45 minutes to an hour for a doctor, it still isn't anything massive comparatively. The patients are getting same day appointments and results which is basically unheard of in the field of medicine. However understandable this is, it is still annoying from the sonographer's perspective to have to wait for the doctors because we are still on a strict schedule that affects other patients and, to be honest, also affects my personal time on some days. If this only happened once in a while it would be one thing, but this is a daily, if not hourly occurrence.

When I finally track down the doctor, he is tied up with another emergency. This is just the way a typical day rolls around here. He ends up doing two things at once, on top of calling the hospital to let them know we have a patient that will be coming over for delivery. Since Anna is late in her pregnancy and her fluid levels are low, he will most likely recommend going ahead with a scheduled c-section, but she must go over to the hospital for monitoring beforehand. I know, this is a lot of information, which is why when I return to the ultrasound room to relay all of this I will try to do it in the simplest way possible. Most couples do not come to ultrasound appointments expecting to get admitted to the hospital immediately afterwards, so I expect this to be an eventful conversation, to say the least.

I walk back into the ultrasound room with a little hesitancy as I know this conversation all too well.

I look at Anna and pause. "The doctor is recommending that you go over to the hospital and prepare for delivery" I say to her.

Anna seems to be slightly shaken by this, but she looks at her husband with tired, aggravated eyes and glances back to address me.

"So does this mean I am having a c-section today?" She questions.

"I am not sure what the final decision will be, but your fluid levels are low enough that we need to monitor you and the baby out of precaution. You are also far enough along that the doctor is recommending delivery. Your baby is breech so a c-section is definitely going to be something that is discussed as soon as you get over to the hospital," I say.

Anna looks bummed out. She sighs, grabs her husband's hand and starts to get up to leave. Most patients will put the safety of the pregnancy first, even if it means changing the birth plan. It naturally just takes time to process and accept these changes and switch to the next path, as with anything.

Before leaving the room Anna turns around and looks at me and asks, "Can we go home to get our bags first? Or stop to get some lunch before heading over?"

Without fail, these questions are asked every single time someone is admitted to the hospital after the ultrasound. The answer is always the same:

"It is recommended, for the safety of you and your baby, that you do not make any stops and just go immediately over to the hospital," I reply as if I have said it a million and a *half* times.

We can't force patients to do something that is recommended, but we can just strongly encourage it. They have to make those decisions for themselves. I sense slight irritation in the room, so I suggest that the partner go pick up the bag and some lunch to bring back to the hospital. This usually quells things for the time being. Anna smiles at me, she still has a very happy, healthy baby regardless of the possible birth plan changes ahead of her. She is disappointed but she isn't devastated.

Once Anna and Adam leave I won't really have any idea

how the rest of her delivery goes. I could write her name down and go look her up at a later date to check on the outcome, but this is where my encounter with this patient ends. It's quite interesting to think about how many different steps there are. I am typically the first and last steps before the little babes make their way earthside.

I sit back in my chair and take a moment to breathe. Not that I truly have a moment, but I have to force myself to take these tiny breaks as often as I can to get through the day. I barely have time to drink water let alone get my reports done. I peer at the digital clock on the bottom of my computer screen and realize I am not as late as I thought I would be for my next patient. Thank God. But the same sound still churns in my head. Tick tock tick tock.

8:59 a.m.

PHEW, WHAT a morning so far, at least nothing has been too serious, I think to myself; I should have knocked on some wood. I have been doing this for too long and I should know better. I've only seen two patients this morning but it already feels like I've run a marathon. I glance down at my Apple watch, precisely what I thought, I have already walked about seven thousand steps and it isn't even close to lunch time. So, that's close to a marathon right? (haha!) I search over my list of patients for the rest of the morning and it seems that my next one is here for a routine fetal survey. This is the same exam that I started my day with. My wrist is already starting to hurt and my shoulder pain has been at an all time high lately. But nonetheless, I carry on and get the job done.

I physically open my eyes wide as if to connect my brain to

staying awake. *Need more coffee.* The ultrasound room is clean and prepped for my next patient, when my co-worker pops in for a quick chat. Perfect timing, as I needed a mini vent session after the first two patients.

"Have you seen the waiting room today?" Sarah asks me as if I haven't been opening that door all morning.

I roll my eyes and jokingly tell her no.

There are two types of sonographers, ones that need to sit in their rooms in silence and ones that need to joke and laugh to get all their stress out. We are obviously the latter as you can see from my previous encounters. Sarah starts to tell me about her first patient and how they drove two hours to get here and didn't leave with a 3D picture and were very mad about it, but that wasn't even the reason they were here in the first place, etc., etc. You get the point. In any career there are always things to vent about, whether it be the management or the staff or the type of coffee that is or *isn't* provided. There is always something to complain about, and the grass is not always greener, maybe a different variety but not greener.

Sarah stays for about five minutes too long and I have to coax her out the door so I can get my next patient. I hear her mumble something as she walks back to her room, but I am too focused on not being any later than I already am to listen. I lock my computer screen and head down the hallway. When I open the waiting room door this time, it is visibly full, almost standing room only. We know how well that goes over in an obstetrics office; correct, not well at all.

"Margaret," I call up towards the ceiling, as I try to avoid eye contact with the upwards of 25 people waiting for their names to be called.

I hear some movement in the back corner and shift my eyes in that direction. Of course, Margaret is here with not only her partner but her parents as well, so that makes a total of five adults, including myself, in the small cubicle that is the ultrasound room. *Deep breaths Cassie, you can do this.* I give a slightly fake smile while holding the door to let them in. I hate holding this contempt so early on in our acquaintance, but there is no need to bring this many people into an ultrasound room for a medical exam.

Margaret and her husband seem filled with positive energy, as they should be. Their smiles beam as we walk down the hallway towards the ultrasound room. I can hear the chatter of the grandparents asking if they are going to find out the sex of the baby and what color they want to paint the nursery. I turn to look in the direction of our room and Margaret's husband is already halfway inside the doorway.

"Is this where I sit?" Her husband asks as he playfully puts his legs in the stirrups on the exam table, I am sure thinking he is hilarious, *eye roll*. I silently sigh to myself and outwardly give a slight chuckle as to acknowledge his joke that I see husbands play every other day. He is doing his best to connect with the female aspect of all of this so I'll give him some credit.

After everyone is settled into their correct seats, Margaret on the exam table, no stirrups needed, and her husband anxiously beside her in the designated chair, I begin my little spiel before every ultrasound.

"I know everyone is excited, but I do need to focus on the images of the baby," I look over at the grandparents, "If both of you could stay on that side of the room please," I say with a slight tone "I would appreciate it very much".

It is beyond difficult to do this extremely detailed ultrasound in the first place, never mind with multiple people peering over my shoulder asking questions and basically breathing down my neck.

This is one of the aspects of ultrasound that I wish the general public understood more. As much as ultrasound is exciting and you get to, hopefully, take home cute pictures of the baby, it is first and foremost a medical examination. You don't see people asking to join in on your x-ray procedures or colonoscopies do you? Exactly. Prenatal ultrasound is just as much a medical procedure as a routine dental cleaning is, so please for the sake of all of us sonographers, limit the amount of guests you bring with you. It truly only makes it more complicated and stressful. I don't want your Aunt Susan asking me what every single white line and gray blob is on the screen. I do not have the time nor the energy to give an ultrasound lesson every hour on the hour. I will tell and show you when the time is right, so hold onto your hats and have some patience.

In all seriousness, I truly understand the special moments that an ultrasound can give parents. Being able to connect with a visual to that little growing human inside of you is something nothing else can create. Thankfully there are more and more businesses opening that solely do ultrasounds for "fun," if you will. They take 3D pictures and cute images, basically a non medical ultrasound. Although there is tons of liability that comes with this, I do still think it is nice to have this option for some patients who really want that extra connection. Preferably, after they have gotten the all clear from their doctors that the baby looks healthy, but that's just me. However cute, there just isn't enough time and energy to give this amount of extra opportunity to each and every patient. Of course, there are exceptions to that and we, sonographers, do our best to accommodate most of the requests we get, but the majority of the time we can't do enough moving and pushing to make the baby turn around. Trust me, we wish we had magic wands we could wave, but alas, we do not.

Now, back to Margaret and her "hilarious" spouse.

The grandparents are kindly standing near the side of the room and Margaret is sitting on the exam table with a cheeky smile. Her husband is casually sitting in the chair next to her. I glance at the computer screen, take some information from Margaret, and head over to the ultrasound machine.

"If you could just tuck those towels into your shirt and in the waistband of your pants, please," I ask to initiate the start of the exam.

I can hear her grandparents small talk as I begin. Like I said before, when I ask patients to pull their pants down to their hip bones, it's like they really didn't know they had hip bones to begin with. Usually they make it just below their belly buttons. Okay, I get it, I don't love other people viewing my midsection either, but the patient is pregnant, this is the only way I am going to see the baby. Also at 20 weeks, even though all the apps and social media influencers tell you that the baby is the size of a banana or that your uterus is at the level of your belly button, the baby is still deep down in between your hips bones, so shimmy that towel down.

"If you could lower the towel just a little more we can get started," I tell Margaret.

I continue to set up the ultrasound machine for my exam.

The entire ultrasound usually takes about an hour to complete. Recall, this is the fetal survey, so the typical anatomical evaluation of the baby to make sure every single organ and bone is normal and in the correct position.

I put gel on the transducer and settle into my position for the start of the exam. I quickly glance over to the grandparents and couple before putting down the probe. All eyes are glued to the patient viewing monitor on the wall behind me, my back facing it. I shake off my shoulder slightly and put the probe on Margaret's pregnant belly. I take an internal calm breath and think about things other than this scan for a moment, as if in a moment of bliss. The days are so busy that I sometimes forget there is an outside world waiting for me at 5:00 p.m., which is still 30 minutes past my actual end of my daily shift; I just add it on now because I know it's inevitable.

I start to move the ultrasound probe around Margaret's belly to get a quick overview of everything. Even before the end of my brief two minute assessment, I know the worst news is looming. My heart starts pounding in my chest. I rapidly scan the faces of Margaret and her family to see if they are seeing what I am, but they are all still happily looking at the viewing monitor. My right hand starts to shake slightly. My hand rarely shakes during ultrasounds, unless I am physically tired from the demands of the job, which usually happens on Friday afternoons or when I find myself in an extremely unfortunate circumstance such as this. I try to deflect as I take multiple images of the placenta and uterus before ultimately needing to image the inevitable. I can start to hear my heartbeat in my ears as I begin to take images of the baby. *Boom, boom, boom.* My breathing gets faster and I can even start to feel a bead of sweat running across my forehead.

In these cases, it is as if nothing else exists. I metaphorically search for that key that just can't be found. There are no words, no pictures, no answers. A situation, such as this, might be one of the worst in a human life. Imagine spending half of a pregnancy excited, happy and blissful to welcome a new life into your arms, and then have those feelings, emotions, and plans you have had for 20 plus weeks or even years, just vanish in a single moment.

I take a few more pictures and video clips to make sure I have captured every single detail that I can for the doctors before taking the probe off of Margaret's belly.

"Is that it, the ultrasound is over?" the grandmother asks as if to indicate she did not fulfill what she came here for.

Even the grandparents suspect this exam has ended too soon. I briefly close my eyes for a moment to regain my thoughts and ultimately decide what the first thing is that I am going to say. I set the ultrasound probe on the side of the machine and start to wipe off Margaret's belly so she can sit up while I deliver this heartbreaking news. One more deep breath, I sit back and look at Margaret and her husband. My body is facing them, but my head wants to be anywhere else.

"I am so sorry, but I do have a very serious concern about your baby," I say with the most empathetic tone possible.

My voice is all over the place and my heart rate skyrockets even higher as I wait for their response. I am looking right into Margaret's eyes when she glances down and then towards her husband. Tears are beginning to well in her eyes.

At first, most patients don't understand what this sentence means. This makes sense, seeing as I have not yet explained the outcome. This is one part of my job that *never* gets any easier. Delivering and then explaining the bad news in several different ways so that each individual patient and their knowledge base can thoroughly comprehend what I am saying. This is the hardest, most heartbreaking part of my day. I wish this happened much less often, but unfortunately these awful events happen daily, especially in a busy prenatal high risk office.

The room grows extremely quiet. Even the grandparents that were once breaking the rules and hovering over my left shoulder have backed away and are no longer asking any questions. Margaret looks at me as if she wants me to explain further, however, in her eyes, I know she understands the meaning behind my tone.

"What concerns do you have?" She asks me with a slight whimper in her voice that was absent only five minutes prior.

My mouth is dry and the metaphorical pain I feel around my heart for her is crushing.

That's the thing they don't tell you about this job. At some point, you will not just be a sonographer, but also a therapist, a provider, a nurse, a social worker, a genetic counselor, a picture taker, a scheduler, an interpreter, and possibly the only support that a patient has in these moments. A prenatal maternal fetal medicine diagnostic medical sonographer wears so many hats that they borderline could pose for the cover of a Dr. Suess book.

There is no training to teach us how to handle the emotional ups and downs that accompany the life or demise of a fetus. Physicians get some training in bereavement and clinical palliative care, but sonographers don't even get one day's worth of related instruction before they hit the ground running at their first job. Maybe some hospitals out there provide this, and bravo to you, but most of the ultrasound programs I have knowledge about do not offer this. I guess it does seem like the hospitals should be the ones to provide this depending on the specialty of the care, but it still completely blows my mind that it is absent in the week-long orientation after being hired. But, maybe, there also isn't enough training that could prepare one for anything like this and it only comes with experience.

Thankfully, Margaret does have her husband and her parents in the room with her so they are able to take on the supportive role to comfort her and drive her home. However, sometimes people don't want their extended family there as it could make devastating news more stressful. I don't think people think about the potential for bad news when they invite the entire family to an ultrasound. Of course, I am glad they don't think of the bad news, as this is rare, but it is not impossible. Please just think about who you want to share this moment with and make sure you're comfortable with the outcome, good or bad, when they are present.

I see the tears in Margaret's eyes and notice her husband gently rubbing her back looking down at the floor.

"I have some concerns about an abnormality with your baby that is not compatible with life outside the womb," I explain.

The moment I say this, the entire room starts to weep. I gently touch Margaret's shoulder as if to say, I am here for you and I am so sorry, and start to stand up. Margret's eyes are red and she is covering her face in the palm of her hands. Her husband has his hand around her shoulders and is doing everything he can not to run out of the room. I glance over to her parents and they are silently holding hands down by their sides. The look in their eyes is one of pure empathetic emotion for their daughter and son in law. The kind of look that just wants to take all the pain away.

At this point all I can do is give them some time.

"I need to go show the doctor the images and then he will come down to discuss everything with you in more detail and answer all of your questions," I say, barely able to get my words out.

I hand Margaret a tissue before turning to my computer. The grandparents make their way over to Margaret and her husband. I hear them say they will wait in the car and will give them some alone time to speak with the doctor. I have so much respect for the grandparents in this situation; thank you for giving Mom and Dad the time and space they need to make some extremely difficult decisions. It is in these moments that I witness humanity at its most vulnerable.

The anomaly that is present with Margaret's baby is called "anencephaly;" this is when a baby does not have a cranial vault and only a partial part of the brain is present. Some people may have heard of this term before or even have known someone who has experienced this or seen it in the news or media. This is a very rare finding, though not rare enough, as I have seen it at least a handful of times in my career. This is one of the most devastating anomalies because it is incompatible with life outside the womb, which means if the patient carries the baby to term, she will have to say goodbye within minutes to hours after it is born. This couple has a lot of hard decisions ahead of them.

As I exit the room I can hear Margaret start to cry hysterically in the background. I shut the door behind me, close my eyes and take a deep breath. I walk into the back room to regain my thoughts. One of my coworkers is back there working on the computer. She looks up and sees my face.

"What happened?" She asks, but she already knows.

She gives me a hug and asks if I am okay. I nod and reach for that small piece of paper that is pinned to our bulletin board. The square paper with a little teardrop in the center. I tape the paper to the outside of my ultrasound room and can still hear the echoes of Margaret's cry down the hall as I search for an available physician. It is in these times of grief that life always seems so fragile, yet so under appreciated. My brain wanders between fears of future children and where I should travel to next in the world as I walk down the hallway. The constant ups and downs of my day definitely take its toll on my emotional and mental health. One could argue both beneficial and detrimental.

Finally, I track down one of the doctors; their reaction after viewing the ultrasound is always the same. They are usually annoyed that they have to deal with the time strain it will put on their schedule but also extremely heartfelt and empathetic about the situation when talking with the patient. You would think it was acting, but to be honest, if we don't put up shields in some way or another, after seeing so much despair and demise, we would all run far, far away from this career. The good days outweigh the bad, thank God, but a large fortress still surrounds our emotions, otherwise we would just be crying all day long, both happy and sad tears.

The doctor reviews my images and confirms the worst. It is in fact anencephaly, which is incompatible with life outside the womb. Just awful and completely unexpected. This anomaly can usually be detected earlier in pregnancy if a patient has an ultrasound around 12-15 weeks along, however, if one is not performed, some cases will go undetected until this anatomy scan. The worst part about this finding is that the rest of the baby is seemingly healthy: the baby is kicking around and active, the heart is strong, and on the inside of the mother the fetus usually does well. It is when the baby joins the world on the outside, that it succumbs to this anomaly.

I walk down the hallway back towards my ultrasound room. Passing all the other rooms as I finally reach mine. The doctor is trailing behind me, anxious and concerned for the patient. I give three light knocks on the door to signal that we are coming back in. As I step into the room I can see how red and swollen Margaret's eyes are, her husband's arm is wrapped around her as he cradles his own head in his other hand. This couple doesn't even know the extent of the news I have delivered to them just moments ago and they are already, understandably devastated and in shock.

The doctor takes the stool from the computer, wheels it over next to Margaret and slightly dips his head.

"I am so sorry I am about to give you some of the worst news you will ever receive in your life" he says.

Margaret glances up from her tissues and tries to listen to everything the doctor is telling her, but I know all too well that in these moments, it is like some information comes in and some just flies right over you. I have seen it multiple times with patients, the doctor explains something and then leaves and the patient immediately asks me a question that was answered five minutes prior. Grief is no joke. It will take hold of you, spin you around, paralyze you, guide you, embrace you, and rock your world all at once.

"Your baby has a very serious anomaly with its brain and skull formation. It will not be able to survive outside of the womb once it is born. This is a devastating finding and I am so sorry to have to give you this news today," the doctor says as he addresses both Margret and her husband.

They both shed silent tears as they listen intently to the doctor as he explains all the details, options, and decisions they will have to face.

I hear Margaret ask one more question, "This isn't my fault right? Like, I didn't cause this to happen?"

I am just gutted, the amount of guilt that we as mothers, fathers, caretakers, etc., carry around with us is heartbreaking. Unfortunately this question is either answered preemptively or asked all too often. I look over at the doctor, he gently places his hand on Margaret's shoulder and confidently tells her, "This is in no way your fault and nothing you did caused this to happen." It is truthfully a random, purely traumatic event. There really are no words or explanations to take the pain away.

The doctor leaves the room and I get ready to put on my next hat of being a therapist for a slight moment. Margaret and her husband slowly gather their things and stand up to leave.

A blank stare is all I can manage to obtain from Margaret as I ask her, "Are you okay to get home?" Thankfully, she does have the support of her husband and her parents, who are outside waiting in the car.

"Yes, I just want to leave," Margaret replies in an honest but calming tone.

"I understand," I tell her as I open the door for them to exit. I show them out the back way so as to not have to walk through a possible waiting room full of smiles and joy.

Standing there, heartbroken for this couple, watching them walk towards the elevator, I think to myself for the fifteenth time this week, why don't we have social workers or grief counselors on staff for these times? It's not like it's a rare event in this office. But, hey who am I, I just work here.

10:31 a.m.

I AM now a solid 31 minutes late for my next patient. No time to process any of what just happened, I need to rush to clean up and get prepped for what's next. The phone on the wall rings. It's the doctor that just spoke with my prior patient.

"Can you get that report done as soon as possible, so we can fax it over to her provider?" He asks in a rushed tone.

"I will have it done in five minutes," I reply with a slight tenseness in my voice.

What I really want to say is, "The report will get done as soon as I am finished with the actual patient, have cleaned my room, and have a second to breathe and recover," but I keep it to myself and hang up the phone. Doctors are stressed beyond belief now more than ever, I get it. But, we are dealing with stress as well and it would be beneficial to all of us if we just communicated that together rather than getting rude and pushy on phone calls or emails.

There is no time in between patients to actually begin to process each individual case. I'm not sure if this is for the better or for the worse. Findings like these can either paralyze you and make you feel like a complete zombie when you're at work. Stripping you of any emotions, leading to constant emotional burnout, and leave you in a state where you go from happy to crying in seconds. This can also lead to a possible imbalance of emotions outside of work, which is never good. From snapping at a spouse or mentally unable to be present, the lifestyle it can create can be detrimental. Leaving work at work is imperative, and I thank the good Lord for the beep on the machine when I clock out for the day.

It is a fine line we walk between being way too overwhelmed and overstimulated by the constant ups and downs of the emotional roller coaster we are on day to day and being able to separate and compartmentalize these events and leave them at work without letting that trickle over into our personal lives. How I can go from seeing multiple miscarriages and losses every day to then go home to my healthy family and be present and active is beyond me. The only way that I get through it is to somewhat tune it out, put up that metaphorical wall without taking on the emotional stress of each patient I see throughout the day. I am certain this way of coping is not unique to this field of work, but in a lot of aspects of medicine and beyond. One patient is healthy and the next is a complete mess. These are the details that do not ever get discussed in school. The programs leave it out, as if it doesn't exist. The real kicker is when you get thrown into these difficult situations and feel blindsided to then find out this is how it has been all along.

As I hang the phone up I am scrolling down to see that my next two patients are here; of course they are. I am already late for my ten o'clock patient and I have one more after her before lunch time. However common this occurrence is, it never gets any less annoying. I always used to wonder, why don't we plan for this and give the schedule a buffer for times like these? But in reality you really can't plan for any of this. It is all completely and utterly unpredictable. Speaking of unpredictability, my phone rings again. This is strange, first of all my phone never rings, and second of all twice in one day is unheard of.

I answer with a slightly skeptical tone, "Hello?" I hear beeping and shuffling on the other line and a couple seconds go by before I hear a reply.

"Hi, Cassie? Can you come over to the hospital room, Stephanie had to leave and I need someone to scan this patient STAT?"

It is one of the doctors over at the hospital suite. I sit in my chair and think for a moment. I lean back with my hand on my forehead. My legs fan out to the sides to try to relax my body before the train that is about to hit.

"I guess so?" I reply as I roll my eyes and try not to sigh too loudly.

At this point I am probably not going to get lunch today which isn't out of the ordinary. I step out of my room to explain the situation to my manager as she grabs my ten o'clock patient, which also isn't convenient, but we have no other choice. Once that is figured out, I start to head over to the hospital. Remember our office is an outpatient facility, but it is connected to the hospital so we do get these calls on occasion to scan patients that are emergent. I just didn't expect this phone call today, right now, at this exact moment.

I walk swiftly through the multiple corridors and parking garages, yes, you read that right, which eventually leads to the ultrasound room at the hospital. I scan my badge too many times at different blocked entrances to make it through multiple different doors before finally reaching my destination. Out of breath with my fitness watch screaming at me, I finally walk into the hospital room. Even before I sit down at the computer to get logged in I hear shuffling feet coming from down the hallway and the voice of one of the resident physicians. I predict they are headed to this room to discuss the emergent case with me; my prediction is correct. Sure enough, as I glance at the door they are quickly making their way inside to update me on the situation.

"Thank you for coming over, there is a patient who needs a dating scan. She just showed up and is currently withdrawing from street drugs. Can we bring her down to you now?" the resident barks before even saying hello to me.

I think her mouth might have also just breathed a little fire as she was speaking so fast. My eyelids are so tired already and I can feel my stomach rumbling with hunger. I have no idea what this patient's name is, what her history is, or how far along in pregnancy she is, but hey I guess sure why not I am totally ready to scan her *right now*.

"Sure, just give me a minute to turn on my machine," I reply without even making eye contact.

Sometimes respect in the corporate hospital world is extinct, not for every situation, but for most. Every single person who is "on the ground working" is overworked, underpaid, and exhausted. That's not even throwing in all that personal life has to offer in those same categories. I have no idea how some people work 20, 30, 40 plus years in this environment. It is truly unstable and would make anyone question their careers at a time or two, or maybe daily in my case. This is not to say that there is any one contributing factor, because there isn't, it's the global view that is off track. The single thing that keeps me coming back every day are the patients; making a difference and saving lives is badass. This is probably true for most of the medical world, I mean who else is going to do it? But, I can only speak for myself. I can sense the stress and exhaustion emanating off of the resident as she verbally relays broken sentences to me. I can physically feel the tiredness inside me and the annoyance in my soul when she is talking. Like I said, there is not one person in medicine who is going to say stress isn't a part of their daily routine.

Why hasn't America figured it out yet? I mean most of the same teachings from 100 years ago in medical school are still being taught today, yet doctors and providers are also expected to stay up-to-date on new protocols and treatments.

I guess the bottom line comes down to change, and change is hard. It is by no means impossible, but it's not a walk in the park either. Whether it's changing the patient flow in a large established office to changing the type of paper towels that are used in the exam rooms, change will drive complaints out of the woodwork. I get it, we all have something to complain about, because let's be honest if we are the ones doing the work shouldn't we be the ones making the decisions? *Wrong again.* We are so far removed from the ivory tower and political decisions it is not even remotely tangible. I am sure some private practices and offices have made strides towards a more fulfilled and commonsensical workplace, but corporate hospitals are nowhere close, which leads to burn out and chaotic, stressful discussions between coworkers and their superiors.

The resident and nurse leave to get the patient as I briefly skim through the bare chart that was provided for me. Not much as far as history for this patient, due to the fact that she has not received care at this hospital previously. As I am halfway through reading about her drug abuse history the nurse wheels the patient in on a wheelchair. The patient appears to be asleep, is half dressed, and attached to a million different IV tubes. I found out through the limited information in her chart that she is assumed to be about 25 weeks pregnant, but has had no prenatal care. Now back in the day this was fairly typical, right? Women would deliver babies at home all the time, and may not even know they were pregnant until later on in the gestation. However, these days this is pretty unheard of. Now, I am all for home birth, water birth, natural birth, whatever kind of birth your heart desires. My only caveat to any decision is a safe birth for both mom and baby. That being said, which I have stated before, this patient is clearly not being safe with her choices during this pregnancy.

In these moments, I always have to take a minute to step back and remember that these patients are struggling, no matter how hard it is to see their side of the pain. Addiction is real, but forgive me if I am naive in any way to the actuality of this affliction. I see it almost daily at this practice, to some extent or another; some women are actively trying to get the help they need and some are going through the detoxification process, such as Olivia, the patient in my room, who is currently in the midst of an addiction crisis.

"Hi, Olivia, my name is Cassie and I am going to be doing your ultrasound today," I say in a caring tone.

I am standing in front of her wheelchair looking directly at her, however her head is down and her eyes are closed. "Is there anything I can do to help you get onto the exam table?" I say as calmly and directly as possible. Olivia doesn't seem to be acknowledging my presence or my question. I see her adjust slightly in the wheelchair, her eyes look lost and the rest of her face looks tired. I can't even begin to imagine what addiction is like. I have witnessed it in some forms personally, but never enough to get a full understanding. This poor girl has her whole life ahead of her, yet here she is overdosing, shaking and about to give birth in the next few months.

Olivia's nurse motions for her to stand up and starts to help lift her onto the exam table. She cries out in what seems like pain or agony; the scream can be heard all the way down the hall. She is in rough shape. I walk over to the other side of her and assist the nurse in getting her on the table. As soon as she is on the table, she lies down in a fetal position and basically goes back to sleep. Not exactly helpful for me, when I need to scan her abdomen. The nurse briefly checks on her and quickly makes her way out the door without so much as minor instructions on what to do if the patient starts to need help, and that, I am definitely not trained for.

I want to dive into that last sentence for a moment. Ultrasound is technically categorized as a clinical job, but we are only clinically trained in basic life support including CPR and first aid. We are not trained to manage someone in a full-blown overdose situation or someone who is in need of more aggressive forms of care. Yes, I can take a blood pressure and have been trained to do it through my previous EMT (emergency medical technician) training. Yes, I can help a patient acutely with vomiting or briefly passing out, however this is not in my written job description provided by the hospital.

So, even minor things such as blood pressures I am not technically allowed to do in my role. The problem is that patients and nurses alike tend to group sonographers into that "clinical" aspect of the patient care team. I am not a nurse, I did not go to nursing school and I have no desire to be a nurse. Nurses think I will be able to handle this patient when they are out of the room, but in reality that is completely out of my scope of practice and really I am not even allowed to be doing anything other than the ultrasound. Hell, the hospital barely lets me transport the patients back to their rooms, never mind perform vital signs. There are rules and protocols for everything even if they make utterly no sense.

That being said, when my patient starts flailing around or asking for more pain medication or vomits I now have no nurse to help. They are supposed to stay with the patient during the exam in this situation, but they are short staffed like every other department these days.

Olivia starts to wince and moan, it looks like she is in pain, but I can't be sure. She is coming down off of an overdose of drugs and her body is not happy about it. The only thing I can liken it to is a hangover and that's probably one tenth of what she is going through physically. Her arms stay tucked into the front of her chest and her body starts to shake pretty heavily. I put my hand on her shoulder and her body seems to calm a bit.

"Can you roll over on your back for me Olivia? This exam will only take a couple minutes and we can get you back to your room," I say as I try to coax her into consent.

Olivia starts to roll over, but her body remains stiff. I

reassure her that this halfway roll is good enough, maybe not for my ergonomics and shoulder pain, but I am able to start my exam nonetheless. I hand her a towel to tuck into her pants. She just lifts up her shirt enough to expose her pregnant belly. Tucking towels in is a feat I don't want to attempt; I think to myself, getting a little bit of ultrasound gel on her pants is the least of her concerns right now.

Olivia is slightly over halfway through her pregnancy. To be honest this gestational age, 25 weeks, is my favorite to scan. The baby is big enough to start seeing little personalized details, but also still small enough for me to evaluate all of the pertinent anatomy. I can already tell visually that she most likely has some extra fluid around the baby. Technically this is diagnosed by measurements, but without those it is already evident. The extra fluid makes it extremely easy to see the baby, thank God, seeing as I have to do arm gymnastics to try to scan Olivia who is barely cooperating for the exam. She keeps falling asleep and turning farther over on her side, making my arm seem that much shorter when I have to constantly reach over her to get my images. I keep asking her to move closer to me on the exam table, but I am not even sure she is awake enough to hear me.

I continue the exam, explaining out loud to Olivia all of the different things I am evaluating on her baby. She basically ignores me the entire time. I get most of the images that I need and end the exam.

As I am about to place the ultrasound probe back on the machine I hear Oliva murmur a question quietly, "Can you tell me if it's a boy or a girl?" Of course, *of course* she wants to know the sex of the baby but could care less about the health of it.

A silent rage comes over me as I take a deep breath and reply, "Of course, it looks like you are having a baby boy, congratulations!" I usually add in the word healthy baby, but in this case the irony is palpable; even though the baby is doing great on the inside, it will be a really tough recovery once he comes out.

I start to clean up Olivia's belly from the ultrasound gel and hand her a couple of printed pictures. She takes them rapidly but then immediately falls back to the bed in the fetal position. Her body still has a slight tremor to it, she looks like she is freezing. I place a warm blanket around her shoulders and start to dial the nurse on the phone. Of course they don't pick up on the first call, and it never gets less frustrating even if I know they are just as short staffed as we are. Finally, she calls me back and says, "I will be right down to get the patient, thank you." While waiting I sit at the computer and start to type my report. I wonder what kind of situation brought

Olivia to this point and how awful and honestly heartbreaking it is to see her like this. All of a sudden she sits up on the exam bed and starts moaning in pain again. She is grabbing at her stomach and tears are streaming down her face. This poor woman. I start to comfort her just as the nurse arrives, thank goodness.

"Why didn't you call us sooner?" Scolds the nurse as she enters the room frantically.

I am sure she heard the moaning down the hall on her way here.

"I did," is all I say in response.

I say goodbye to Olivia and wish her good luck and the nurse is out the door with her wheelchair before I can say anything else. Probably for the best.

At this point I am so exhausted mentally that I can barely remember how my morning went. From one patient to the next there are such drastic changes that my mind cannot possibly make sense of in one day.

I sit down at the computer to finish my report and hopefully have time to clock out for lunch. That's right, again with the time clock, clocking in and out for lunch is also mandatory. As if there weren't enough rules in the medical field, they also have control over how many extra minutes, if any, we get for lunch and to reset our brains for the afternoon. The computer screen is so bright, I glance over to the time in the bottom right hand corner. Alas, 11:41 p.m. My 11 o'clock patient is most likely still waiting for me to return. That will leave just enough time to rush back over to the office, scan her quickly and without any issues, grab half my lunch out of the fridge, heat it up in the microwave for four minutes and shove it down my throat, all before my next patient. I metaphorically wipe sweat off my brow.

The medical field is no joke. There is no stopping, literally none. The second I clock out for the day I try to erase all the emotional memories and trauma from the day so that I can recuperate for the next, nevermind the rest of the week ahead. As if there is any recuperation from this career. Our shoulders, necks, and wrists are all already broken and injured. According to a survey published in the Journal of Diagnostic Medical Sonography by the Society of Diagnostic Medical Sonography and Sound Ergonomics LLC, almost 90 percent of sonographers scan in pain daily. This is one of the most high risk ergonomic jobs there is in the medical field. I don't think most people understand the physical demands associated with ultrasound. It is so important to teach proper practices in school and abide by ergonomic rules within ultrasound departments. The employee health system is not even trained well enough to educate and deal with the risks that come with hiring sonographers. We are indeed a liability, but also an extremely necessary piece of the healthcare puzzle.

I would love it if a group or an individual took it upon themselves to start some kind of wellness company that went around to hospitals and properly educated them about the needs and limitations of these types of careers. It seems that those in careers associated with radiation exposure get the proper training and assistance from hospitals, but when it comes to little old ultrasound we just get shoved to the discard bin.

I cannot count on one hand the amount of times I have been discharged from employee health, just to return a month later with the same injury. It is about prevention, not the "clean up after the mess has already happened" approach. This method has failed miserably for decades and something needs to be done. So, that being said, yes sonographers need a hiring package that includes massages, stretching routines, gym memberships, and physical therapy visits on a monthly basis. Not every medical career needs these specifics, it will change from position to position and be individualized, but it *needs* to happen. This is an enormous piece that is missing from modern day medicine, the piece about caring for employees on a more holistic level, not just a financial level. I promise we will all be happier, stay in the field longer, and be willing to help out way more. This will also in turn save each and every institution thousands if not millions of dollars every year on employee health visits. I've seen the data and it's astounding. Please someone take this on and change the culture of working in medicine on a global level. I'm begging you.

I clean up my ultrasound room, turn off the machine and proceed to head back over to the outpatient office.

Once getting back I quickly log into the computer in my out patient room and search frantically for the patient's name that has been waiting. Thankfully she only just got here about 15 minutes ago. Patients being late is also not a rare occurrence, but how can we blame them when we are constantly running behind schedule as well? Things happen, life happens.

11:52 a.m.

MY SCREEN looks blurrier than it has all day or maybe my eyes are just tired. I can feel the impending headache start to loom. I let my eyes close while I finish typing the last of my report from the previous patient and envision my head hitting the pillow. A nice restful sleep is all I need, even 20 minutes just to get through the rest of the day, I think to myself. Not going to happen, but it was nice to day dream; sometimes just the visual is all I need. But today, today I need full blown hibernation.

Scrolling down to the middle of my computer screen I see Chelsea, my next patient in the queue. I glance at the bottom right hand corner and notice the time. Chelsea is scheduled today for an ultrasound for something termed "decreased fetal movements." This is a general term used to describe a wide range of maternal experiences when the fetus is not active.

Maybe the fetus is not normally as active at a certain time of day or maybe Mom is complaining of not having felt the baby move in hours. For either of these cases, I never take this indication lightly. I *loathe* this indication. My blood pressure elevates when reading through her notes. "Patient called, the baby has not had typical movements today, adding on for ultrasound this afternoon." My heart quickens as I immediately stand up and rush to clean my room. I don't want this patient waiting any longer to make sure her baby is not in danger.

I head back down the hallway, nearly falling through the waiting room door and call, "Chelsea" into the waves of bobbing heads.

A woman with long dark hair stands up and casually makes her way over to me. She looks like she is going to deliver any day now. She holds her hand on the nape of her lower arched back and her waddle is more than noticeable. She is smiling and sleeping at the same time. The end of pregnancy is exhausting. Chelsea is at about 38 weeks, only two more weeks, give or take, to go. Her partner is slowly trailing behind her making sure nothing was left behind. He offers to hold the door as Chelsea and I walk through. We make it all the way back to my room, but not before Chelsea slips into the bathroom next door. Her husband, Steve, sits down in the chair opposite me and smiles. His eyes wide and his heart so ready to love on this little babe as soon as possible.

"Has Chelsea mentioned the baby not moving much today?" I ask him while typing notes into my computer.

"She said that she just isn't as active, but did feel her kick slightly this morning," he says.

I look up at him while he continues, "She tried drinking juice and changing positions but the little one just seems cozy in there I guess."

I feel a knot tighten in my stomach. It gets tighter and tighter with each bit of information he is giving me. Chelsea returns from the restroom and sits down. She lets out an enormous sigh. I turn my attention to Chelsea now, and ask,

"Have you had any complications with your pregnancy?"

She blinks as if to think before replying, "Nope, everything has been great aside from the pretty much constant morning nausea."

"That can be rough," I say, keeping the conversation open ended in case there was any other information she forgot.

My thumb presses the button to lift the exam table into the correct position and Chelsea situates herself appropriately for the scan. My mind is racing. Not just before this scan, but literally before every scan that I perform. It is such a gamble, what am I going to find as soon as I place the camera down? With my history and my job description, it is not always a normal healthy baby, as we have seen throughout my day thus far. The sheer enormity of how many different things I could see is overwhelming. I focus back to positive thinking. Usually with decreased fetal movements the baby is just in a weird position, or they changed positions from their normal spot which makes the movements harder to detect.

Chelsea and Steve are both focused on the patient viewing monitor on the wall behind me. She looks tired and he looks eager. Her, ready for a nap and him, ready for any slight bit of connection with his unborn daughter. My right hand reaches for the transducer and I take a deep breath before placing it down on her belly.

For some reason I start down low on her abdomen, I don't look for the heart beat first, like I normally do, I immediately image what is down low in Chelsea's pelvis. A bright white circular area shows up on the screen, the baby's head. "Baby is head down," I say in a monotone voice. My visual clues and intuition start to kick in. The baby isn't moving. There is way too much amniotic fluid around this baby. The umbilical cord is not pulsating. My heart starts to pound. I feel dizzy. This is all happening in mere seconds. I move the camera slightly higher and try to get an image of the beating heart, but fail. I take the camera and angle it all over Chelsea's belly in hopes of finding the right spot to where I can see a viable heartbeat.

I fail again. I feel like I am going to pass out, but I take a silent breath and continue. Chelsea and Steve are staring at the screen clueless to my internal reactions thus far. I need to be certain of what I am seeing before I say anything to them. I take the transducer and image up at the top of her uterus, lots and lots of amniotic fluid.

"Aww I think I just saw her kick!" Steve says into the stress laden air.

My heart just shatters into a million pieces. I want to cry, I want to scream. Instead, I calmly take a few more images to confirm the worst. I do not see the heart beating. I do not see the baby moving. This is a demise so severe that it takes me a minute to gather my thoughts. Why am I the one who has to break this news to them? Why didn't I get training for this? Where is my reference guide on how to handle a situation like this? In reality, there is none. This type of despair does not have a manual. This type of despair is only communicated through sheer empathy and strength. No matter how many times this has happened in my career, every time feels like the first. My mouth is dry and my swallowing is audible in the silence of the room. The anxiety that resides inside me is palpable at this point.

Chelsea turns to me and asks, "Is everything okay?"

I don't answer immediately and finish taking the rest of

my images. Once finished I set the probe down and begin to search my brain for the words to use to relay an impossible result. Chelsea and her husband are on edge now, sitting up and both staring at me looking for the relief that will not come.

"I am so sorry, I do not see the heart beating. I am so sorry I have to give you this news. Your baby has passed away," I manage to get out but not without my eyes starting to water. I blink fast as if I am not allowed to feel any emotion.

Chelsea and Steve stare at the ground and then Chelsea screams "Nooooo!" Her wailing is loud. It is a cavernous guttural scream from deep within her soul. Steve is holding her but his reaction matches the tune of her mourning.

I truly never know quite what to do in these situations. Every single person and couple is different. It is my job to adjust my delivery depending on each individual case. This isn't easy and I don't always get it right, but hell if I don't give it my best shot.

"So there is nothing you can do?" Chelsea whimpers in between her sobs.

"I am so sorry, there is nothing we can do," I say.

"I am going to go get the doctor and you can ask him any other questions you might have."

"We don't have any other questions," Steve says, "we just

want our baby back."

"I understand and I am so deeply sorry for your loss" I leave them with this before saying "I am going to give you a few minutes and I will be right back."

In these late demise situations, it is literally just hit after hit of bad news. First you get the news of no heartbeat, then it's the news of, well, you have to deliver the baby anyway, oh yeah and if it doesn't work with induction then you will always have a c-section scar to remind you of the pain you endured. The *worst*. Completely unimaginable, yet Chelsea and Steve are not alone in their grieving. Whether it happens right before delivery or even at delivery, such in the case of a stillborn, this does happen. This is a risk we all take when bringing life into this world. It is the saddest and worst thing ever and I wish there was a magic medicine to take this risk away for everyone. But, of course there is not. Life is risky, no matter what version of it you are in. The most powerful things I have witnessed are parents such as Chelsea and Steve or any others out there that go through a tragedy like this and then try and do it all over again in hopes of a different outcome. That kind of strength is unmatched.

A teardrop paper is not needed on my door to signify a loss. The entire office can hear Chelsea's screams. I quickly walk to the doctor's office to inform him of the results. He hangs his head and closes his eyes as if to say an internal prayer for the family. He immediately gets up from his desk and follows me back to the room. I knock on the door, a little louder than usual and we quickly step back inside. Chelsea and Steve's eyes are bloodshot and there is a whole mountain of tissues on the ground. Steve looks like he is going to throw up. The doctor lets out a sigh and expresses his condolences.

"The next steps are not going to be easy. They are going to suck, to put it bluntly," he says to them.

He continues explaining what to do next, although I doubt any of it is being received. Chelsea needs to head over to the hospital. Steve needs to be her support system and his own in the same breath. He finds whatever strength he has left and helps her up off the table and out the door. The hallway is quiet, open, and ready for them. Luckily it is lunch time and no other patients are roaming the hallways with their viable baby bellies in view. Chelsea and Steve can exit without any more hardship. In times like this, there are no words, literally nothing I can do or say to comfort or help the situation. I can't even fathom putting myself in their shoes, yet they are not alone. They exit the back door and even after the door closes far behind me I can still hear her wails in the back of my head.

After sending them on their way, I need a minute to compose myself. Not just a minute, I need an hour to decompress from this situation. My schedule does not allow for a minute, never mind an hour. I don't feel like eating, I don't feel like talking, so I just sit down at my computer, shut my door and breathe. A text vibrates on my phone. I glance at the screen, it's from my husband. "How's your day going?" It reads. How do I even relay an answer to this? Good, bad, stressful, horrific, humbling, all of the above? I guess that's it, all of the above.

12:41 p.m.

ONCE I decide to go to the lunch room there are about three other employees waiting to heat up their lunches. Who in their right mind thought it was a good idea for a 50 plus staff office to only have two microwaves and let everyone have lunch at the same time is beyond me. But, then again a lot of the corporate decisions behind non-profit medicine baffles me on a daily basis, as you can probably tell by now.

I hear the beeping of the microwave and finish washing my hands in the bathroom next door. Finally, it is my turn to heat up my food and sit down for ten minutes to eat. Some days I choose to eat in my ultrasound room by myself; today is definitely one of those days. The constant human communication can sometimes take its toll and I just need to sit with my own thoughts for a bit before continuing the cycle for the afternoon. Don't get me wrong, being able to have the outlet of socialization in my career is one of the added benefits of ultrasound, but every once in a while you need some peace and quiet with yourself to reflect.

After being in this field for nearly ten years I have not seen it all, but I have seen and heard a lot. So much of this world now is based on social media experiences and an unrealistic view of the world in general. From TV shows to the smart phone in your pocket, I am sure that you have a preconceived view of ultrasound and what the sonographers actually are doing during the exam. Most of what we do is not portrayed in the media. Just like other areas of medicine that are glamorized on television. Lots of what we do is sacred.

All areas of medicine are practiced differently, even if medical school tries to encompass it all in a short four years. Yes, medical students go on to residency programs and specialize, but there is nothing like hands-on experience. No textbook or lecture hall is going to prepare you for the real world of medicine. I am here to tell you that ultrasound is not immune to this aspect. There is a recommended and required way to perform exams and there is also just performing an exam. There is a medically indicated exam and there is a 3D keepsake imaging appointment. There is the way the female anatomy looks in a textbook and there is the way it actually looks either under ultrasound or during a pelvic exam. Ultrasound has so many different aspects that are not even discussed in school.

I have now taken multiple different board examinations to do what I do. To be as specialized as we all are working in prenatal MFM ultrasound, we usually have to sit for close to five board exams. We study each individual part of the body from the small tissues in the fetal brain and heart to the maternal growing uterus and placenta. Each exam is about three hours long, if my memory serves me correctly, and I have no idea how many questions but a lot. I have a lot of opinions, let's say, on the process of these examinations. First of all, when you walk through the door of the building it feels like you are in an airport. They basically think you have textbooks strapped to your chests and notes tattooed on your arms. You must walk through a metal detector and basically strip down to your skivvies to prove you're not packing notes. I wasn't even allowed to have a hair tie on my wrist when I walked into the testing room. I mean I get the safety of certain things, but my goodness if I wanted to cheat that bad I shouldn't be spending upwards of $300 on a test that really doesn't even determine my scanning skills.

As far as the images on the test, it's like they are from 50 years ago when ultrasound was first invented for medicine.

In hindsight this is probably for the best as it does force you to really know what you are looking at, as the ultrasound machines nowadays are extremely high tech and give a much better image. But, still I thought I was good at sorting through the multiple shades of gray, black, and white, until seeing the poor quality of the images on the tests. Granted, I took my tests years ago so they could have improved, but I doubt it.

The other interesting thing about these exams is the questions they ask about patient diagnoses. I mean, our title is Registered Diagnostic Medical Sonographer. However, once you get to the clinical world the first thing you are always told is "you are not diagnosing, just describing what you see." So, in order to become a sonographer I need to know exactly how to diagnose and take a test on it but then in practice I don't do any of that. Hmm, seems suspect to me.

However crazy and backwards this sounds, it actually is all in good reason. We are specifically trained and tested on diagnosing so that we can give the physicians exactly what they need. We are diagnosing, not just picture taking. What we are *not* doing is explaining in detail and following through with the care of the patient after the ultrasound. This, my friends, is for the doctors to do, but some, most, days it also may be temporarily written into my job description.

If we don't image it and don't see it then the doctor won't, simple as that. If I don't image that mass in your liver or the clubbed foot on the baby then the doctor will never know it existed. This is the reason for the multiple exams we take, and this is the reason we are so sensitive to the misunderstanding of ultrasound and the sonographer's role in general.

I am not just the picture taker, I am also the person who diagnoses, communicates with you, and keeps you calm during your exam. I am the one who is checking on your well being as I am imaging your fetus, some days feeling like I have six eyes and four arms. I am the person who relays any good or bad news to you. I am the one who images the tumor that the doctor then takes out in surgery. I am the one who sees the sex of your baby for the first time. I am the one who sees the cardiac defect of your baby and images all the small vessels and structures to be able to discuss with the doctor what the diagnosed defect is. I am the one who initially comforts you in times of despair. I am the one who congratulates you when you are here without any support. I am the one who answers your first questions when they are bound to come up during any exam. I am the one who simultaneously is able to have a conversation with you about something totally unrelated to your exam all while imaging every single organ and bone in your baby's body. I am counting fingers and toes, number of vertebrae, measuring each limb and brain structure to confirm they are all within normal limits. I am looking at your maternal anatomy such as the uterus, placenta, and cervix to make sure they are all healthy and normal during your pregnancy. If I don't see or image the mass in your baby's abdomen or the low amniotic fluid that is surrounding your baby then the doctor is not going to be able to properly diagnose and treat you.

Ultrasound is no joke; it is such an important profession and I feel like the reputation it has gotten over the years has made it seem very misunderstood. Aside from pregnancy, ultrasound can do numerous other things, from musculoskeletal imaging to adult brain transcranial imaging. The world of ultrasound is growing rapidly, mostly because it does not involve radiation, so it is a much safer option for most things. I mean really ultrasound is used for just about everything in the human body. There are even ultrasound cameras that go down the throat to look at organs; pretty fascinating.

I make my way back to my ultrasound room and close the door behind me. These rooms feel like dungeons or basements. The walls are bare, without much character and the floors might as well be concrete. There are no windows and the low lighting makes me want to fall asleep. I barely feel like eating today. It has been a hectic, stressful, and emotional day so far, not that that is unusual, but hunger hasn't been my top priority today.

I sit at my computer and start to zone out for what feels like two minutes, but ends up being 20. I hear a knock on my door. I shake off my current sleepy zoned out state and open the ultrasound room door. It's my manager.

"Hey, it's 1:10 p.m. and your next patient is waiting, is everything okay?" She asks.

God, it's like a babysitter, someone is always watching over me and making sure I am doing exactly what I am supposed to do at every waking second while I am at work. I mean, yes, thank you for reminding me that it's time to go back to scanning patients and fending off the wolves but could there be a little less micromanagement?

"Yes, everything is fine, I just got a late lunch. I'll be right out," I reply with the fakest smile known to man.

Thankfully I am on the other side of the curtain and my face is not visible. Sometimes I just want to scream out loud and let it all out just to feel better before the second half of the day. Between the emotional and physical toll of the patient load and detailed exams and the stressful, chaotic atmosphere inside this work environment, it's a surprise I don't hear more screaming from coworkers on a daily basis.

I remember one morning my friend and fellow sonographer, Jane and I actually sat in my car for ten minutes before entering the building for our shift and just cried, literally cried. There might also have been some light screaming, but there were definitely tears shed. Is this normal? Do people do this before shifts at work? No, this can't be normal, I mean truly it seems rather insane. But, alas we show up day after day, shift after shift and do it all over again.

1:11 p.m.

AFTER MY manager rudely interrupted my much needed alone time, I realize that she is probably right and I do need to get my next patient started, seeing as I am running late once again. Not that the usual happenings of my late nature are due to my day dreaming, just rightfully earned breaks, but I probably shouldn't enhance the tardiness.

I sit back in my chair and start to type in my endless passwords in order to access the patient schedule. I mean I get it, patient privacy and safety and all but sometimes it feels like they are hiding some deep dark secrets in here. Maybe it's a metaphor for some other aspect of the healthcare field? Nah, now I am just overthinking again.

Sometimes just looking at the schedule on the screen makes me anxious. The multiple lines of patients, one after the other, row by row of pertinent and non pertinent information just staring back at me as if it is all supposed to make sense. Honestly, it looks like a puzzle that is impossible to solve.

The reality is just that, time after time, manager after manager has tried to solve the ongoing issues surrounding the office politics or the messy patient schedule and all have failed. The healthcare system in general is flawed, but throw in some incompetent management and it's a recipe for disaster.

In just ultrasound alone we see upwards of eighty to ninety patients per day. Scrolling through the list of patients is enough to make anyone go dizzy.

I click the screen to separate the schedule by ultrasound room to make my list slightly less daunting. My next patient is here for a routine dating and viability scan. This type of ultrasound is performed to assess an early pregnancy for viability and achieve accurate dating information. Typically the patient presents with a last period date and this is how we estimate about how far along they are. Then, once the ultrasound is performed we will either confirm or change the dating depending on what we see and measure. Seems more complicated than it is, trust me.

Although, I have had patients in the past argue with me about the dating of their pregnancy. I mean I'm sorry but the measurements don't lie, maybe you do, to your spouse, but the ultrasound machine and the images are extremely faithful. Science versus memory, hmm I will take science for 1000 Alex.

I had a patient once who I scanned and she was so adamant that her date of conception was correct that she asked me if her baby had growth restriction at six weeks of pregnancy. Now, if you are in the healthcare field or in the career of ultrasound you know this accusation is insane. Growth restriction doesn't typically occur until well into the second trimester, if it's caught that early at all. A six week embryo is the size of a grain of rice, literally, not even a centimeter long. Hence the term embryo and not fetus. Anyway, this patient was visibly angry with me when I told her how far along she was measuring by ultrasound. According to the patient, she should have been nine weeks along, however the ultrasound clearly showed that she was only six weeks. Early pregnancy ultrasounds are extremely accurate, therefore a six week pregnancy compared to a nine week pregnancy not only measures differently it also looks extremely different to the eye. A trained eye knows this fact and obviously my eyes are more than trained for this than hers.

I remember the patient asking to speak to my manager and questioning everything. My manager and I could tell something was up, whether it be infidelity or just a true denial of scientific results. Either way the angry patient went on her way and I will never know the ending of her story. That's the thing about prenatal ultrasound, I always want to know the whole story, but only rarely do I get to follow a patient from conception to birth and forward. There are so many different hands in the pot. The gynecological team before pregnancy, the prenatal team during pregnancy, and the pediatric team after birth. As much of a "specialty" that I am in, it still gets more and more specialized as the needs get more and more complicated. The fact about pregnancy is that no matter the issue or the time constraints, you will always be seen, no matter what. Pregnancy is time sensitive, a short nine months of time. The very concept of waiting months to be seen is metaphorically unheard of in the field of prenatal care; you're pregnant now but you will not be soon. If you and your baby need to be seen you will be seen, no matter what the schedule allows for. This is probably one of the main reasons why what I do is so stressful yet no one addresses the elephant in the room.

One eye-opening aspect about first trimester ultrasounds is that you never know what you are going to see. You could see twins, triplets, conjoined twins, a pregnancy failure, ectopic pregnancy, or sadly nothing at all. The moment twins are identified or even before pregnancy if the mother has diabetes these cases are automatically labeled high-risk and they become patients of the maternal fetal medicine group. The moment that the first image is displayed on the screen during a first trimester ultrasound, that determines the immediate fate of that particular pregnancy.

I gather my senses and start to evaluate the patient's chart that I am about to scan. Just as I thought, the referring provider has not included any of the information that I need; well I guess I will have to just go completely old school and ask the patient when she gets into the room. It is almost as if this form of normal communication ceases to exist in the present world. I constantly evoke the right to ask my patient questions when their referring provider fails to send over the correct records or orders. What? Can the patient not tell you themselves? Is it only accurate information when it comes from the provider that asked the patient the same exact questions last week? The medical field is so backwards sometimes. The way the system and insurance companies require certain things to be done in a certain order baffles me daily.

I start to make my way back to the waiting room doors for what feels like the 500th time today. The door feels heavier as I push it open to welcome my patient.

"Lisa," I call out to the ten full seats in the waiting room.

Thankfully only one woman and her spouse stand up. I hate having to explain that this is an internal ultrasound when eight people stand up and then sit back down the second I mention the word vagina. It's almost as if humans in general forget the way that another human comes into this world is usually through the vaginal canal, so it's not that out of the ordinary to be doing some sort of vaginal exam during pregnancy. But, then again I don't think high school health class has been updated in years, at least according to my assessment of women's health knowledge on the female genitourinary system.

Lisa makes her way to the door with the biggest smile on her face, her husband in tow beside her, hand in hand. The joy and excitement is palpable from this couple. Although I try to avoid most emotions during the work day, sometimes I can't help but join in on the excitement, I mean it is nice to be joyful once in a while at work, right?

Lisa and her husband follow me, blissfully and maybe in a slightly ignorant state, to the ultrasound room.

I enter the room, but first look back around to ask Lisa, "Do you need to use the restroom before the exam?"

She quickly declines the offer but funnily enough her husband accepts and slips into the bathroom before I can give him a hard time. This happens way too often for me not to chuckle a bit under my breath as I show Lisa to the exam table. When he returns, I joke with him saying "Lisa's bladder is supposed to be the full one not yours." He lets out a nervous laugh and sits down in the seat next to her.

Things are about to get somewhat interesting.

I face Lisa and start to give her the instructions for the exam: "This is a vaginal ultrasound, have you ever had one of those before?" I ask, but she is staring at me like she is looking right through me.

Her eyes start to widen and glaze over as if she doesn't understand anything I am saying to her. The pause of silence before she replies "no" is unmistakable. She chuckles and covers her mouth with a little nervous undertone. This is common and to be expected; I mean if you have never had an internal ultrasound it sounds like the worst thing in the world, but if you have had one you know they are the furthest thing from a big deal, hell I dare to say even easier than a speculum exam. But anything is better than a speculum exam, am I right? For all the women reading this you get where I am coming from.

"It is very similar to when you have an exam at the gynecologist. I will need you to undress from the waist down only; you can leave your socks on and cover up with this sheet and take a seat back on the exam table," I say to her after she has overcome the initial shock of the words "internal" and "ultrasound" in the same sentence.

It's true, in the movies or television shows, the ultrasound is pretty much always portrayed as an over the abdomen exam in pregnancy. So, why would women have any other expectation of it? I will admit, recently I have seen it included more, thankfully giving more of a real life insight to women's health and pregnancy, but nonetheless, still extremely far from accurate.

"Only take off your pants and underpants, leave your top on," I repeat to the patient before leaving the room to allow her to change.

I cannot express how many times I have left the room only to reenter to a patient who is completely naked, pulling the sheet up to their neck trying to cover their entire body with a five by five foot, 20 thread count sheet so they don't feel exposed. I mean, I get it, you're nervous and maybe weren't listening to me when I gave instructions, twice, but what the actual hell do you think we are doing to look at your pregnancy? Do you think your breasts need to be exposed to look at your uterus? Dang, so many questions I have in these moments. But again, no judgment, just curious what goes through the patient's brain when this happens. I mean to be honest most of the time it's due to a language barrier and that is totally understandable, but when it's not I have *many* questions.

I close the door behind me and wait impatiently in the hallway. *The hallway.* This specific hallway.

I start to sort of lose sense of where I am and drift off in thought for but a moment, or at least for what feels like a moment. The hallway that I am standing in has seen so many different emotions. It's a sort of spiritual experience every time that I take a minute to step back and think about it. From sorrow to elation the range is vast.

In medicine there are multiple spaces like this that encompass a sort of holding zone, just like waiting rooms, for this invisible and ever changing energy. Although the energy is not always palpable it is always there in some form or another. Even when I am working the weekends and I stroll though, past the multiple ultrasound doors and exam rooms, the energy of what could be or has been never fades. There is a quiet feeling and overwhelming calmness which is the extreme opposite of the chaotic weekday hustle that exists within these walls, but the knowing, just the knowledge of the realities resonate and feel heavy. It is extremely noticeable the difference between the two, which only provides more insight to the importance of this simple yet complicated structure. I mean it is after all just a hallway.

My coworker nudges past me giving me a side eye, sort of breaking my trance of internal thought. Shit, how long have I been metaphorically holding up this wall? I tap a quick knock on the outside of the door before entering, although I am sure by now she could have gotten dressed and undressed ten times.

"Are you all set?" I ask through the pulled curtain separating the hallway door from the exam table.

"Yes, I think so," Lisa replies in an uncertain voice.

I pull back the curtain only to slip to the other side. Lisa's husband has a wrinkle forming above his brow and is staring at the floor. Lisa is sitting patiently on the exam table, with her top on, thankfully.

I start to raise the table so that it is ergonomically positioned to my ultrasound machine. Insert another dad joke here: "Going up," Lisa's husband says with a sly look on his face as they chuckle together nervously.

The next five minutes hold a special place in my frustrations. Not with the patient, but with women's health in general. The relationship that women have with their body has been tarnished over many years, from social acceptance to social media, none of it has shed a positive tone on women knowing their own bodies and being proud of them. I mean come on, we grow and birth children, let's not forget this enormous feat.

Also, any type of internal procedure is going to be awkward and an invasion of personal space. I have always been taught in school and in clinical rotations to allow the patient to guide the ultrasound probe into the vaginal canal herself, or to at least offer this first. Some women will not be comfortable with it and that's totally fine, but the offer should be there. I find it extremely wrong when some women express to me that with previous internal ultrasounds, if they have had them, they have not been given the offer to guide it themselves. I don't know, this just seems inconsiderate, due to several different circumstances such as prior trauma or just extreme genital sensitivity. I understand it is a medical procedure, but who knows your body better than yourself?

Well, that's exactly it, lots of women are not told how to know or accept your own body. There are so many women who know nothing about their bodies, and that is directly related to our culture in America. We, as a country, are so uncomfortable with even saying words like vagina and penis and sex, that the community at large does not receive crucial information about their own organs. It's no wonder patients come in for a vaginal ultrasound and have no idea what I am talking about. We must teach ourselves or rely on family and friends to educate us enough so that we feel confident. Does that make any sense? I don't even remember health class teaching me anything other than how to put on a condom. Sounds familiar in American society, am I right? Teach the temporary solution rather than prevention? How many of you, at high school age, were basically handed condoms or birth control and told "here take this" or "wear this, you don't want to get pregnant" instead of being taught how our bodies actually work and letting us decide for ourselves what the right course of action might be? I could go on and on about this, but the bottom line is this: teach women about their bodies, everything, not just the easy things, teach us about the good, the bad, the ugly, I promise it will be better that way for everyone.

I position my ultrasound machine and stand at the foot of the exam table. I motion to the stirrups.

"You can place your feet here when you are ready," I say to Lisa, although I know she most likely will never be ready.

Lisa does as I request, however she is still basically sitting on the headrest of the exam table and her big toe is barely touching each of the stirrups. Even if a patient has had 40 pap smears or internal exams in their lifetime, they will never scoot down to the edge of the table enough for the exam. I will admit I even fail to make it to the correct position during my own appointments. I mean come on, I do this for a living, but even my body rejects the awkward, awful position that stirrups put us in. It just is not instinctual for us to want to be hanging off an exam table with our legs spread; why would it be?

I pause and take a silent breath and calmly ask, "Could you please scoot down about six more inches until your bum is at the end of the table?" Lisa laughs and scoots down, although not completely enough, it will do for the beginning of the exam. I will take what I can get at each step of this process, as it might seem like second nature for me but for her it is a complete unknown.

It never ceases to amaze me all the different ways that women try to reach to guide the ultrasound probe into their vagina. Some bring their hands in front of their abdomens, some in back of their legs, while others look like they are in a complete pretzel. I feel like all natural instinct goes out the window when you are nervous and your private space is being invaded, so it is understandable, however wild, that our brains do this. Most of us lose all common sense in the face of fear and uncertainty. Well, I think that's actually a known phenomenon that has been studied for years, but nonetheless.

I squeeze some sterile gel onto the tip of the ultrasound probe and pass it under the sheet in between Lisa's legs.

"I am going to pass this to you under the sheet for you to guide in," I say as I wait for her to take over under the paper sheet.

Lisa consents that she is comfortable to guide the probe herself. She seems confused so I show her the ultrasound probe which has a sterile cover on it with some sterile gel on the outside for comfort. I use my fingers in a pinching motion to show her the length of the probe that will actually be inserted in the vagina, about one fourth of the actual transducer. The probe itself is longer so that I have a handle to hold on to once it's inserted.*

After I have explained the insertion instructions to Lisa she puts her hand under the sheet and reaches for the probe. I find her hand and place the handle within her reach. I gently hold on to the other end while she positions it comfortably. Once she is ready I take over and demonstrate the side to side, back and forth motion that I will be doing during the exam. She agrees that this is fine and we move forward with the exam.

When I start an early obstetrics scan, I always prepare by telling the patient that I will need to look around first and get oriented with their anatomy before I tell them anything. The reality is that we as sonographers do relay the results of this early ultrasound, which is basically telling each family what they have been waiting two to three months for, if there is a heartbeat or not. Sometimes people even get the surprise of their lives when we find two or more heartbeats. These moments sometimes make me feel like I also have two heartbeats, stressed yet excited all in one.

---

* I have personally had quite a few internal ultrasounds and I can say from experience they are nothing compared to what you expect, which is the response of the majority of patients.

The first image appears on my ultrasound screen and I briefly peek over at Lisa, her eyes shift over to mine and her husband's are fixed on the viewing monitor straight ahead. In these moments, and truly in any moment leading up to delivering previously unknown information, the patients are searching my face for clues. Is she going to smile, frown, laugh? Will this give insight into the results of this ultrasound? These are some of the questions that are running through a patient's brain before I give the first words of hope or utter devastation.

As I move the ultrasound transducer slightly higher to the top of the uterus I can see the pregnancy. I start to scan and sweep through the entire uterus and my eyes do a double take, pun intended. I see two pregnancies. My heart starts to beat a little faster and my brain works a little harder as I try to navigate and organize images on the screen. I change a few settings and start to zoom in to assess for heartbeats.

At this point both Lisa and her husband are still oblivious, at least that's my assumption, because neither of them are screaming, crying, or questioning me yet. Usually if there is a patient that can somewhat tell what's going on on the screen, they will start either drilling me with questions or scream so loud that it makes me jump. As soon as I see the two pregnancies I turn to scan both her and her husband's faces, nothing. Okay, I think to myself, let me just make sure I am seeing two heartbeats and make sense of everything before I deliver the news to this couple. I remember my first time delivering the news of surprise twins. I thought I was going to pass out, my heart was racing so fast. Even though this news had nothing to do with me, my autonomic response took over my brain. Another reason why this job is way more than just pressing buttons and taking pictures.

Now that I am sure of what I am seeing and have all the information I start to talk about the findings. I briefly look in the direction of Lisa and her husband and place a light touch on the outside of her knee with my left hand.

"I see a pregnancy inside your uterus," I say while pointing at the flickering grain of rice on the screen. "See this right here, that's the heart beating," I say as I start to scan to the other heartbeat "and see right here, this is a second heartbeat, you're having twins!" I finish as I wait for the response.

Lisa lets out a primal screaming sound and throws her hands over her mouth in shock.

"No fucking way!" is all I hear from Lisa. Her husband is laughing with his head in his hands.

"I'm sorry I didn't mean to swear, I just can't even believe this," Lisa says while her whole body is basically jumping up and down on the exam table.

The image on my screen follows her excitement as it shifts

up and down, side to side with her movements. I let her and her partner rejoice in this surprise news for a minute before continuing the ultrasound.

Lisa lets out a deep breath and says, "Okay, I don't think this shock is ever going to wear off, so please show us everything."

I start to image the first baby. I use my multiple settings on the machine to get a heart rate, 145 beats per minute, very normal. I scan over to get the heart rate of the second baby, 135 beats per minute, also completely normal. Sometimes when I am delivering this information it is almost as if the parents assume the heart rates will be exactly the same, like they are sharing a heart, but this is far from the case, unless they are conjoined twins which these two are not, thank God. I have seen conjoined twins a handful of times and those are extremely difficult cases to navigate.

Lisa's husband Derek, turns to me and asks, "Can you hear the heartbeat?"

This question is asked in almost every early ultrasound appointment I have had and the reality is this: it is not recommended by any ultrasound or prenatal accrediting body to be listening to the fetus's heartbeat at this early gestational age with ultrasound. Period. You may have seen it performed in TV shows, or had a friend who's doctor did it, but this is not the standard of care. I was taught in school, as all schools should teach, that it is not routine care to use this tool during a viable early ultrasound. That being said, I do not want to scare you, ultrasound is completely safe, but as in any imaging modality we use the ALARA (as low as reasonably achievable) principle. This ensures the safety of you and your fetus under the tested and studied areas of ultrasound. Basically just trust us, just like you trust your CT tech or X-ray tech; we know what we are doing to keep you and your baby safe. I went to school to do this and that means I am a trained professional. Maybe the TV shows and movies out there should be doing a little more field research as to what is actually happening before falsely representing us. *There I said it.*

"We do not listen under ultrasound, but at your ten to twelve week visit with your provider they will try to get a Doppler tone with a handheld device that will let you hear it," I answer to Lisa's husband Derek who is clearly still shaken up by the news of twins.

He is switching positions from standing to sitting like he is doing some sort of gym work out. The dimples on his cheeks are deepened by his ever lasting smile as he continues to look back and forth from the patient viewing monitor to Lisa. Now that the news is slightly settling in with her I can start imaging again. Her body is not bouncing up and down with her breathing and my screen is still again. I finish up with multiple pictures and measurements, of course double the work for double the baby. I make sure to print a lot of pictures and I always try to get at least one picture that has both of the babies in the same photo, because they will grow fast and this may be the last time that happens.

"I am all done, I'm going to take the probe out and bring the table down," I say as I press the button with my non-ultrasound hand to move the exam table back to the floor and remove the vaginal probe with my other.

I swear we need like four hands to do ultrasound, but that *also* wasn't in the job description.

There are different types of twin pregnancies, but this particular type is pretty cool, because it's basically like two singleton pregnancies developing simultaneously in the same uterus. Each came from a different egg and has its own "house" so to speak within the uterus. They do not share anything except the space of the womb. I could go on and on about the vast information there is here as it relates to twinning, but I appreciate not everyone is as enthusiastic about embryology as I am. The amount of events that need to happen at exactly the right time even just to make one pregnancy exist is extraordinary, never mind doing it twice, and at the same time.

Lisa gets dressed behind the curtain and I can hear her and

her husband's smiles as if they could make sound. I can also feel the potential stress in the room and the amount of questions they are going to have going forward. Unfortunately for them this is not the room to start that conversation, but fortunate for me. The pictures I printed for them cascade down from Lisa's hand almost to the floor. Hey, like I said before, double the baby, double everything else, literally, and this is only the start.

My fingers are still shaking from the exciting news and slight adrenaline rush that comes with delivering the news of twins. I am using the delete key a little bit more often while typing up Lisa's report, giving them a little extra time to swoon over the news is always a good thing.

Lisa has an appointment with one of the providers after her ultrasound today, which makes it easier for me to defer all of her questions to her visit with the doctor. That's another unique thing about this practice. We see ultrasound patients from all over the state and sometimes the country. High risk, normal, and even some out of state patients that are on vacation. The majority of our cases are high risk, which is why our hallways serve the most unique of cases. But, we also see routine pregnancies as well, so don't let the warning sign on the front office door fool you.

I leave Lisa and her husband to bathe in the bliss and fear

that are twins and head down the hall to track down one of the medical assistants. Technically, we are supposed to follow the rules and put the patient back in the waiting room, just to wait for another room to open up, but I like to press my luck and check in before doing so. Usually this works in my favor and I can just bring the patient right to their next appointment, no hassle, no waiting.

Unfortunately for me it is Monday and the hallway is a ghost town, due to everyone being busy in exam rooms. Monday's in the outpatient medical field are insane. Between employee vacation time, the already busy schedule, and the constant add ons from the weekend, Monday's might be the busiest day of the week, other than Friday's. They may be neck and neck for the win.

I strike out at my usual routine, so I head back down the hallway towards my room. The door to my room is slightly ajar as I step inside.

"Lisa had to use the restroom again," Derek says as I make my way into the room.

"No problem, when she is back I am going to have you two sit back in the waiting room until the provider is ready," I say as Lisa walks back into the room.

I walk Lisa and her husband to the waiting room. As I open the door to let them through my eyes glaze over with the amount of other patients that are sitting there waiting for their names to be called. I squint from the glorious afternoon sun that is shining through the bay windows on the other-side of the room. I shut the door and head back to my dungeon room. Damn you, Monday.

1:36 p.m.

MY PREVIOUS exam took slightly longer than intended, simply due to the fact that again, double the baby double the work. I am now six minutes behind for my next patient; I'm surprised it's not more. I inhale a deep breath through my nose, close my eyes and exhale through my mouth. This no windows thing is really getting to me today. I need some vitamin D to bring some energy back into my body. My eyes open to my computer screen and scan down the schedule to the next patient's chart.

I can feel the rage start to boil up from my esophagus, or is that heartburn? Either way, I am angry. Of course, they booked a case that should be an hour long in a half hour long spot. Of course they did, because who cares about the sonographer and if she might want to get out of work on time today or save her shoulder from pain? I swear nothing we propose as a protocol ever gets put into action, it's just a soft suggestion that we stick to the schedule and times allowed. Patients can show up whenever they want, say whatever they want, act however they want and yet we will still bow down to them as if they are the kings and queens. Okay, that was a little dramatic, but you get my point. We still have lives outside of work. Not that this particular scheduling flub had anything to do with the patient, this is totally our bad, but my sidetracked mind lumps all of it into one basket. Oh healthcare, how organized it all is... I think to myself as my eyes hit the back of my skull for the *millionth* time today.

Even though I know this particular patient is going to take upwards of 60 minutes or longer, she is only booked in a 30 minute slot, which means one of two things: either I am going to get out late again today, or I will have to make up the time with another patient scanning with lighting speed. It is usually the first case scenario, and I am pretty much over never getting out on time. Especially today, I just want to go home and rest my brain and my shoulder.

I reign in my emotions and angst and wrap them up into an invisible ball, metaphorically throwing it out the non existent window. I need to focus, this next exam is going to be a tough one, both physically and mentally. I glance at the time on my computer screen and can feel the anxiety bubbling back up my throat. God damnit, is there a limit on how many Tums you can take in a day?

My hands hover over the keyboard as I click through the patient's chart. I was the first person to scan her a week ago and I remember it like it was yesterday. I mean it was only two days ago that I got the follow up information that the mass I found was cancerous and she now has been diagnosed with lymphoma at 28 weeks pregnant. Ironically enough it was in this exact same room. Shivers run down my spine. I can't imagine bringing her back into this room after what transpired during her initial prenatal ultrasound last week, but there are no other rooms available so this is our only option.

Last week Mary was here, with me. She was sent from an outside practice for a scan. She had been complaining of pain under her belly button and had a couple other minor risk factors that were concerning. She is a little older than average for pregnancy and has chronic hypertension (high blood pressure) throughout her gestation. Her referring physician thought it would be a good idea to have her seen with us. Little did we all know what we were going to find.

I remember scanning Mary and analyzing her uterus and fetus. Everything looked perfect with her baby, the placenta, and the uterus. I know that one cause for concern with the amount of pain she was in was her placenta. The doctors wanted to make sure there was nothing going on, such as an internal bleed or the placenta not attaching correctly to the uterus (also known as a placental abruption).

Like I said, everything with the fetus and uterus looked great. I remember as I started to scan up towards her area of pain, that's when I spotted something that seemed off. I have done hundreds if not thousands of scans like this one: a patient is sent with a specific area of pain and nothing is ever found other than a muscle tear or ligaments that are merely stretching during pregnancy. But, unfortunately for Mary, there was a much bigger and much rarer finding.

As I continued to scan, I remember seeing a large oblong area right underneath the belly button region of Mary's abdomen. I remember physically scrunching my forehead and almost audibly saying "hmm." Thankfully no noise came out of my mouth and Mary did not glance up at my face at that exact moment, but I was definitely unsure of exactly what I was looking at. I rarely find anything to correlate to minor pain that patients experience; however, this seemed, based on a gut feeling, more concerning.

Usually scanning over the belly button can cause lots of shadowing on the image, due to the air that is between the ultrasound probe and the skin, but this did not look like an air shadow. I continued to image the unknown area, taking all sorts of pictures and measurements from different angles and areas on her abdomen. I added images of the blood flow to the mass and even some small videos for the doctor to review. Based on my experience, it sort of looked like a hernia, which is a small protrusion of bowel. This is a relatively common finding in adults that can cause pain and discomfort. It had the same sonographic characteristics as a hernia does so I figured this could easily be in the differential diagnosis.

After reviewing everything with the doctor and showing him the images, we walked back to talk to Mary about the results. I had even convinced the doctor that this could be a possible hernia. I remember our conversation vividly and exactly what the doctor said to Mary. He told her he thought it could be a bowel hernia, but to be on the safe side he wanted to get more imaging, such as an MRI just to make sure; thank God he did. Bowel is extremely difficult for ultrasound to assess with accuracy. Sure, we use it here and there but it is not the gold standard by any means. MRI is a great resource in pregnancy because it does not expose the fetus to any unnecessary radiation.

Mary went and got the MRI three days later. Two days after that the results came back. This was no hernia. Mary had full blown lymphoma. The mass we were seeing in her abdomen was a mass secondary to the lymphoma. Now, this is extremely rare, but I can't get over the fact that if 41 year old Mary hadn't gotten pregnant, she may have never known about this until it was too late. To put it not so lightly at all, this baby saved her damned life.

The growing pregnancy and the hormones flowing through her system put pressure on the disease which inflicted symptoms. This may have never been the case if Mary was not pregnant and she may not have found the cancer in time to get the treatment she needed. That being said, as much as this new finding of cancer is as brutal as it gets, especially during pregnancy, it was truly a blessing in the ugliest disguise imaginable.

Mary has now planned to start chemotherapy treatments next week. She is here today to assess the fetus and uterus again. Now, this is not the typical course of treatment. Most of the time women choose to wait until after delivery to start therapy, but Mary had no choice, her condition was aggressive and if she is going to survive long enough to deliver this baby and parent it she had to take action now, at least that's what I read in the oncology doctor's recommendation. She has apparently accepted this fate and returned faithfully to all of her scheduled appointments. She is back today and I can't believe, as coincidence has it, we will be together again.

The memory of her initial visit strains my brain as I take

a deep breath to clear away any of the extra negative energy before retrieving her from the waiting room.

I open the door and even before I call her name I can see Mary sitting off to the right hand side of the room, which is still full of multiple patients waiting for their names to be called. For the brief moment before her name leaves my mouth I notice her hair. She has already fully embraced her current and future destiny. She has shaved her head in preparation for her battle. It was as if she wanted to have some say in this war and God dammit if she can't take control of something. The strength in her eyes is already far beyond any measure of what I have ever personally experienced. How honored I am to witness such pure vulnerability and ascendancy.

"Mary," I call, in a voice that tries to convey all that I am feeling for her.

It feels more intimate, more real, then if I was to call a random person who I have never met before. Her story seeps through my thoughts like a sponge as I hold the door open for her. Mary stands up with the smallest glint in her eye and the corners of her mouth tilted upwards, but no teeth to be seen. A halfway smile of sorts, a controlled smile. Who wouldn't command control when you are in two completely uncontrollable situations simultaneously? Pregnancy and cancer cannot be tamed easily. Some medical journals and articles have gone as far as comparing pregnancy to cancer cells in some obscure aspects. No, but seriously, look it up; it has been discussed in more scientific terms.

I lead Mary down the hallway once again, repeating my path. I am tempted to check my steps on my watch, but decide against it.

"I am just going to pop into the restroom before the exam," I hear Mary faintly say behind me, as we get closer to the ultrasound room.

"No problem, we are in this room when you are ready," I reply, then I turn to look at her with a caring smile.

I actually feel in my bones the empathy I have for this woman. The energy courses through me as I step into the room. I prepare the table with a sheet and towel and wait for Mary. She is here alone, as she was the previous time. I never ask too much about any one person's story, unless they invite me into it with a conversation. But, I am always curious, sometimes concocting fictional stories of them in my head. Without confirmation, Mary enters the room a couple minutes later, anonymously, except for her name and date of birth.

Mary sits down on the exam table and prepares herself. Towels tucked in and the proper directions followed. I start to lift my transducer over Mary's belly and my brain can't help but think about what was found just last week. Now that she has established care with oncology, it's not part of the scan to assess the cancerous mass in her abdomen. My sole focus now needs to be on her unborn baby and uterus. As I spread the warm ultrasound gel over her belly with the probe, I glance over at Mary for what feels like a lifetime, but is actually less than a second. This middle aged woman, seemingly could be at the end of her life, time will only tell. Simultaneously, she is also carrying the beginning of life within her. How much more vast yet short can the universe feel at this moment? I shake off the feeling.

"Could we try to get a glimpse of the little one's face today?" Mary asks in the most respectful and kind way.

"Yes, I am going to try to get you as many pictures as I can of him, he is actually super busy in there and cooperating like a champ!"

Just as I finish my sentence the little stinker turns over and decides that he is only going to show me his spine. Typical, the second I mention cooperation they always do the opposite. Truly their full personalities flourishing even at the earliest age.

The least I can do for Mary is give her as much connection with her baby as possible during this exam. The way I can do this is by pointing out various anatomical parts and giving her pictures to take home. I simultaneously scan to check the wellbeing of her and the fetus, making the exam seem light hearted, fun, loving, and meaningful. I mean this is her baby after all. The black and white two dimensional, textbook like images take away from reality at times, which is both a relief and hardship. In this case, a hardship. I try to get a 3D image of the baby's face but he just does not want to give it up. I instruct Mary to move around side to side a bit, at her comfort level, but he decides today is not his day for photos. I wouldn't normally try this hard for extra pictures, but I think everyone can agree that the circumstances warrant this extra time.

The exam is finished, everything looks perfect, even the stubbornness of the fetus is reassuring. Mary wipes off the gel and starts to stand up. Her legs retreat from under her and she sits back down rather abruptly.

"Are you okay?" I quickly ask, as I place my hand on her right shoulder. She braces herself on either side of her hips on the table and begins to stand again.

"Yes, I got this," she grunts with a smile. At this moment I didn't know I needed her strength, but I did. Witnessing the strength of these mothers over the years has accumulated within the corners of my brain and has been kept for safekeeping. If she can do this, then shit, I should be able to at least get through this shift, right? It gives me a sudden burst of energy as Mary exits the room and is on her way. Funny isn't it? The energy shift from the moment I recognized her name on the schedule to the end of the exam. I watch her as she turns down the hallway and out of sight, internally wishing her well; this could very well be our last encounter together.

The two o'clock hour during the work day is always so dreadful, am I right? What is it about two o'clock that feels like the day is never going to end, why didn't it feel like that at eight o'clock or even lunch time for that matter? The afternoon yearn for hibernation hits hard today. My eyelids feel heavy and the dim lights in my room only encourage the matter. Coffee, I need coffee, but I barely have time to pee, never mind make myself a coffee. I choose to empty my bladder instead of filling it with more diuretic liquid before clicking on my next patient. Does it make sense that sometimes I literally am running to the bathroom? Like physically running, using the facilities as quickly as possible and then running back to my room, because I am so behind on the schedule. Most days I want to just scream or cry of frustration at this point. I have had enough for one day, but then I summon the strength I just witnessed from Mary, close my eyes and take a deep breath. In through the nose, out through the mouth. Repeat three more times.

2:02 p.m.

M Y EYES open and focus on the middle of my computer screen. If only the palm tree laden desktop background could be my reality for even a second, I think to myself. It feels nice to sit down for a minute and just be, pretending the everlasting schedule doesn't exist. Pretending to feel the warm breeze as if it's drifting off the image.

There is never any "down" time at this office, and if there is, you better believe you should be cleaning, stocking, organizing, or hiding in the bathroom, because someone from management will be speaking to you otherwise and calling you unproductive. The micromanaging atmosphere that healthcare breeds is not sustainable, hence why the average annual turnover rate is about 32%. If that statistic isn't eye opening to the huge changes that need to be made within the healthcare industry, then I don't know what is.

To put that into perspective, if we have about 50 sonographers on staff and we lost 32% that would be 16 positions per year. On average it takes about six months to a year to train a new employee for this position, so I'll let you do the math as to what that cost versus benefit analysis is, but trust me, it isn't good.

Shaking off the numbers and statistics my mind reroutes to the next patient chart. I hover the mouse over the patient's name and click the icon. In the distance I can hear the click clack of one of the nurses and her shoes coming down the hall, that can only mean one thing: an add on patient. I quickly hustle to gather any pertinent information about my next patient, thankfully I am only about ten minutes behind as of right now, but still behind nonetheless so hopefully I will not be asked to take the add on, on top of my schedule.

When add on patients are necessary it is a slight nightmare, as the schedule is not built to allow such time for this, which makes no sense, but hey who am I? Apparently a minor part in the scheduling solution as a sonographer that works this process every damned day. All of our multiple suggestions are placed ever so delicately on a table for later once again.

Turns out my next patient is here from an outside facility, so per usual I do not have much information. I gather the gist of what I do have. Her name is Susan, she is here for a reassessment of fetal growth due to suspected intrauterine growth restriction. This basically means the baby was measuring small at another office and she got sent to the high risk office for a second opinion and recommendations if it does indeed turn out that the baby is smaller than expected. There is so much more knowledge and information I could divulge into here but I will save you the biometry lesson for now.

I spin in my chair and head for the exit to my room. As I enter the hallway of ultrasound rooms my eyes and my brain track each door, back and forth like a zig zag across space. In one room a patient and her partner are leaving with smiles on their faces and a long string of ultrasound pictures. In another room with the door shut I have no visual of the ongoing exam, however I can hear the wailing of tears and heartache as they echo through the hall.

As I make the turn to the waiting room there are multiple patients waiting at the checkout to book their next appointments, nurses are taking vital signs on patients in the little alcove of the hallway, and phones are heard ringing off the hook. This place is a zoo. There is not one ounce of calm energy floating around, it is all chaotic. Not really the type of energy that a patient needs when being referred to a high risk clinic. But, the words high-risk and calm don't usually make it onto the same page.

Hopeful I can bring some sort of peace to this next patient, I open the waiting room door and call "Susan" at a slightly louder than usual tone.

Through the bustle of the room, a shorter than average, kind looking lady stands up and starts making her way over to me. She is here alone, which is not out of the ordinary and to be honest, like I have alluded to previously, quite the relief, at least for me. The smile on her face tells me she is not stressed in the slightest. She makes eye contact with me and smiles as I hold the door for her to enter. I smile back, although mine is a much more strained smile. As we turn the corner back towards the ultrasound room I can barely hear her behind me. I look back just to make sure she is still there.

With her presence confirmed, we walk into the ultrasound room. Now that we are inside the room with the door closed, her facial expression and tone of her body changes. She is sitting on the edge of the table and her smile is only half as wide as before. Her eyes look scared. I sit down and turn towards her.

"Hi, Susan, my name is Cassie and I will be doing your ultrasound today," I say.

"Can you tell me why your doctor's office sent you here

today?" I ask.

Susan looks slightly confused, as to say *shouldn't you already know why I am here*? Yes, this is true, however I always like to hear it in the patient's own words, because the game of telephone is dangerous in healthcare.

"I had an ultrasound at my local hospital and they said that the baby was measuring small," Susan explains.

"They didn't really give me any more information, they just sent me here for a reassessment."

Interesting, I think to myself, because the notes I have read about this patient say exactly the same thing. Usually there is some sort of miscommunication, but it seems so far we are doing pretty good.

"Great, thank you for that information. I will be doing a complete assessment of your baby again today, including lots of measurements. I have here that you are about 32 weeks along, does that sound accurate?" I ask her.

"Yes, 32 weeks and two days today," she replies.

Again, I usually start my scans the same exact way every time, but for some reason, again, I choose an alternate route. Maybe my brain was sick of gliding down the same groove hour after hour, or maybe my intuition and instinct kicked in unknowingly. My eyes are drawn to the head area. The round skull, with its bright white bones and internal black and gray patterns seems strange. Just not quite normal, not completely abnormal, but not normal. I couldn't put my finger on it, until I started to put measurements from side to side and around the complete circumference of the cranium. The head of this fetus appeared much larger than the rest of the body. I have been doing this long enough that even subtle differences hit me like a ton of bricks.

Ultrasound is as much a visual assessment as it is a data driven evaluation. I can visually tell what gestational age a fetus is, how much amniotic fluid is around the baby, and any gross anatomical abnormalities with just my naked eye. I don't need official measurements or data points to tell me everything I need to know. Something is going on with Susan's unborn baby, I just don't know what yet.

I continue my investigation as I scan up to the chest area and abdomen. The heart seems to look normal so far. I scan through the left and the right chambers respectively. Something still feels off about this view, so I add some additional measurements that are not typically taken with routine assessments. As I calculate the cardio-thoracic ratio my brow furrows and my mouth starts to twitch to one side. I usually try to hide all of my external physical expressions so as to not alarm the patient, but I am an open book right now. I glance over to Susan and she is not looking at me, thankfully, but she is staring at the patient viewing monitor with a questionable look on her face. I am not sure if she is confused at merely what she is looking at on the screen or if she is able to decipher the measurements and is deducting a conclusion of her own.

No words are exchanged between Susan and me for a good eight minutes. I continue my thorough exam, measuring each and every bone and body part that will give me a detailed report for the doctor.

Susan finally glances over to me and asks, "Does everything look okay?" *This question.*

This falsely categorized, simple question. It might be the only question that I dread answering and truthfully never really know how to answer. Every time a patient asks me this, I never know what to say. I fumble through my internal catalog of words and responses in my brain and finally respond with some sort of word vomit that never feels right.

"I just need to get a few more pictures and measurements and then we will go over everything," I reply in a voice that *definitely* tells her something is wrong.

Even when patients ask me this and everything does look "okay" I hesitate on what to respond with. Because unfortunately I know all too well that everything can look great one day and the next it could all come crashing down.

This puts an ambiguous nature to pregnancy outcomes, but isn't that the gamble we all take anyway, with anything in life? We just obviously never want to think about that when it's gambling with a human being, even if the good outcome outweighs the risk 9.9 times out of 10. Like I said, the only reason I constantly see the 0.1% is because I work at the only high risk prenatal hospital in the state. Another data driven reason, not my favorite, but worth the explanation.

Susan looks over at me and I can see now that she is trying desperately to read my face. I stay as statuesque and poker faced as possible. My eyes do not meet hers as she glances over, I keep scanning and clicking away at my machine. When I look at my screen after measuring the femur, the upper leg bone, I can tell something in my face changes, but my reaction time is too slow. I can't control the pursing of my lips and downward tilt to my mouth that happens as I read the numbers on the screen. In my periphery I see Susan still staring at me in hopes of reading my mind. She is well aware that the next thing I say to her is not going to be "everything is looking okay."

I always internally start to panic when I find things that are not normal and even more so when they are extremely abnormal. You would think after the hundreds of times that I have given out bad news, my immediate body reaction would not tend to fight or flight mode, but it always does. Maybe it is my own past trauma that spikes this response or maybe it's only human. But, then I think about all the humans working in the Emergency Departments and Paramedic units out there. They are constantly faced with unimaginable acute challenges; does this mean they are consistently in fight or flight as well? I then think to myself, there is usually one difference, at least between frantic emergency care and the care I am giving. The patient that I am treating has no idea what is going on, literally not even an inkling of a paper cut, before I hit them with possibly the worst news of their lives. At least patients in an emergent state are either out of it or are well aware something is going on, even if they are scared shitless. Withholding knowledge that is going to change the trajectory of someone's life in an acute way is tantamount to torture. I know something is wrong and is going to change everything, and I am the one to drop this bombshell.

I finish taking all the images that I need, as well as all the measurements. In this case my measurement screen is double the length as typical, due to the nature of the abnormal findings. Not that Susan will be able to notice this minor change, but my mind always wonders what each patient will pick up on, because it is always something, but never the same something.

"You can clean off the gel on your abdomen with this towel

and sit up when you are ready," I say to Susan, delaying the inevitable.

I can feel my heart skip a beat before I quickly decide how to break the news. I place my transducer down in the curated slot on the machine and turn towards Susan, looking her straight in the eyes. I feel my chest, *lub dub*, another skipped beat.

"I do have some concerns about the measurements that I took today of your baby. I know part of the reason why you were sent here was to assess this. I am going to go review these with the doctor and we will be right back to go over everything with you and answer all of your questions in just a few minutes." I strategically say my words as if they are scripted.

I hate that though, saying partially scripted lines, as if these patients are not human. I understand all the legalities and such, but come on, if chivalry is not completely dead yet, then neither is being frank. Susan looks at me like I have three heads. Her eyes seem to be looking at me but are actually staring over my right shoulder at the wall. She hasn't said anything in about 30 seconds and I am beginning to wonder if she heard me.

Just before I start to repeat myself Susan sighs and says, "So what does that mean?"

She clearly needed a moment for her working brain to

catch up with her worried brain. Those two together make a mad combination so I understand taking a minute to sort a few things out.

She is now looking directly at me and her face has changed from scared to brave in a moment's time. It is extraordinary to witness all of this on a day to day basis. Not that I am consciously acknowledging it at the moment, but my reflection on it does remind me of how remarkable it is. How remarkable humans, mothers, and fathers alike are. How resilient we can be, even given the worst kinds of news.

Susan presses on: "What kind of concerns do you have?"

I can never get the doctor in the room fast enough after I drop the "concerns" bomb. I always contemplate not saying anything and just running down the hallway to get the doctor before the patient even notices I am gone. Who am I kidding, the patients notice everything, especially when it involves their unborn baby, who wouldn't?

"My concerns are about the growth of your baby, and the measurements that I took today. Let me just go get the doctor. I am so sorry that I have to tell you all this, but I promise he will go over everything with you shortly," I say sincerely.

I truly am sorry and I truly am worried for her and her baby. This isn't easy, none of it is. Not even a "normal" pregnancy is easy, so I can't imagine one with question marks, at least not personally. Professionally I see it everyday.

Susan takes my reply and decides it's enough for now. With the promise of a doctor in the near future, it usually is. I tell Susan not to panic if it takes a little while for me to return, I am just waiting for the doctor to finish with a prior patient before he is available. I tell her where the restroom is if she needs it and back out of the room.

Sometimes patients think they need to hold it all together in front of me; however, as soon as I shut the door behind me I can hear the wails of sorrow and dread. I don't hear any of this from Susan, at least not yet. She has proven to be a very stoic lady thus far, making her a little harder to read than most, but I believe she is just waiting to have all the information before engaging in any sort of emotion. Now that is something I wish I could teach myself.

My first stop is to the back room where we keep our extra computers for reporting. If I don't have all my measurements exactly in order and all my images labeled correctly then I may as well not even find the doctor. He won't even give me a moment of his time without all of the pertinent information and to be quite honest, I wouldn't if I was in his shoes either. Fifteen calculations later and I finally have a completed report. Isn't this what computers are supposed to do for you? But, then again I guess I did go to school for this so, throw up that Doctor Evil pinkie finger, those thousands of dollars did add up to something.

After I meticulously comb through my finalized report I walk down the hall to the bay of doctors' offices. The reading physician for today is on the phone so I stand outside his office until I can hear the click of the receiver signaling he is finished. These waiting times are what the daily schedule does not take into account. The unexpected happenings that apparently the ones who manage the schedule do not think happen but literally *always* do. Again, zero proactivity in regards to healthcare systems and their management.

I hold up the wall for five long minutes before he finally ends the call. As soon as he does I make my presence known by stepping into his door frame in plain view. I don't want him taking another call before he talks to my patient. He does not acknowledge me in the slightest. I look at him and wait, outwardly patient and inwardly annoyed, for him to address me. I glance at the clock on the back wall, 2:59 p.m.; damn going to be late again I think to myself.

Finally, with his eyes still glued to the screen in front of him, he says, "Cassie, what do you have for me?"

These interactions never cease to amaze me. I mean, look, I get it we are all overworked and busy, but can we just remember we are in the same sinking ship and help each other out?

I step forward and start, "I have a patient sent from an outside facility, question of growth restriction. It looks like all of the long bones are measuring extremely small and the head is larger than gestational age."

There is a pause between my words while he looks over all of the images and the measurement that I am presenting to him.

"This isn't good, dammit this sucks for this patient," he says bluntly.

Okay good, I think to myself, at least he still has a heart.

"Alright, let's go talk to her, '' he says as he stands up, throws his headset off and is already halfway down the hallway.

I open the door to enter the ultrasound room and there is Susan, sitting on the edge of her seat, her hands clasped together on her lap. Now that I think about it, her belly barely looks pregnant. I know what the doctor is about to say to her and looking at Susan just makes my heart ache. Her entire world is about to change. The doctor takes the stool on wheels and sits down in front of her. He introduces himself and tells her that he wants to discuss the results of the scan with her.

"I do have a concern about the growth of your baby, it is somewhat asymmetrical and quite a bit less than expected for the age of your pregnancy," he continues.

"So what does that mean?" Susan replies.

He straightens himself out and clears his throat before replying,

"It means one of two things. Your baby could have a lethal skeletal dysplasia or it could be a normal variant."

Can you imagine? Basically being told that your baby could either be sort of normal or not survive outside the womb; but we don't know yet so we can't tell her one way or the other. I try to summon the strength I witnessed with my previous patient and will it into Susan through the air. I look at her, her eyes are glazed over and she is staring at the floor in front of us.

The room is silent for a beat and then Susan says, "So, what do I do?"

"First, we would want to get another growth scan of your baby in about two weeks, and then we may have a better idea of what is going on," the doctor replies.

"So basically you are either saying that I am carrying a little person who may be quite a bit smaller than average or there is some sort of problem that he will not survive when he is born?" She asks.

The doctor just nods his head. At this point I can see Susan is starting to get teary eyed and I hand her a tissue. The conversation carries on as I just stand at the computer screen pretending to be busy. I am basically just there for support of both Susan and the doctor. For Susan, handing her tissues and as a confidant and for the doctor as his right hand man, well woman in this case.

The amount of grace, confidence, and maternal instinct that this woman already possesses is utterly inspiring. The gist of her conversation with the doctor is Susan being more worried about the life this child will lead in the future, rather than the unexpectedness of an abnormality. She is extremely worried about bullies in schools and how people may treat a human that may not be of "normal" appearance. The one thing I do notice is that she is constantly apologizing for either crying, asking too many questions, or for simply just stating her concerns. Nothing that one should ever be apologizing for, especially after the news she was just given. I turn towards her and say, "Susan, there is nothing to apologize for, you are simply just being a mom." This woman is already a mother, just listen to her. Her valid concerns about quality of life and more. She looks at me, tears in her eyes again, and smiles. Thanking me silently for my sincerity.

Every single interaction in my day is different. From happy, sad, exciting, and devastating to angry, worried, and frustrated. I go up just to come back down an hour later and then an hour after that I could be spinning in circles. Thankfully the one thing that I can stay grounded in is time.

As much as I am going through all of these journeys with each of these patients, I also know there is an ending to it. There is a point in which the story changes from one person to another and I can recover, even if it's minimally. My reflection on this brings out the actuality, whereas my acute experience tends to be more chaotic and, at times, dramatic. This career isn't for the faint of heart, as cliché as that is. This is likely why the turnover rates are so high. It takes a lot of active energy to separate my story from all of the patients' lives in my day to day schedule.

After the doctor and Susan leave my room to schedule her follow up growth scan, I close the door behind me and sit down. I can feel the weight of that last hour expand in my chest and almost fall through my body as I sit heavily in the chair. My head tilted back and my arms slumped to either side. A metaphorical and actual vision of exhaustion. The day is nearly finished, do I dare look at my schedule to see how far behind I am? Do I dare look at the time? Almost as soon as I think it my eyes dart over to the bottom right hand corner of the desktop. 3:32 p.m., 32 minutes late for my next patient. I had high hopes that my last encounter went a lot quicker than it actually did, but alas my hourly tardiness is never ending.

3:36 p.m.

I HEAVE my body back into an upright position and begin the same repetitive task of researching my next patient. So far it seems that this will just be a routine growth exam.

Please let this be an extremely normal routine case, I say to myself almost out loud. I am not sure if my body and my brain can hack another complicated venture.

Tanya is scheduled at 36 weeks of pregnancy because she is what the medical world likes to call "advanced maternal age." The insurance world, however, likes to call it a "geriatric pregnancy." How fun, I can't wait to be 35 or older and be labeled geriatric already (eye roll). Of course, this is only when someone is pregnant, but still, how rude. Some accrediting body made the decision that pregnancies when the mother is 35 years of age or older are now considered high risk. This being the case, we usually see them for an appointment during the third trimester to check on growth, fluid, and the wellbeing of the baby. My patient, Tanya, is scheduled today for exactly that. No other notes about some extra abnormal finding, just a simple growth scan.

Even though I am assuming this will be a normal exam, the fact that I am still 36 minutes late taking her into my room heightens my stress levels. Do you see the pattern yet? The stress does not leave the building. Well, that is until I go home and can't get the events of the day out of my head.

The waiting room is still packed like a jar of pickles when I open the door.

"Tanya," I call into the never-ending abyss.

A woman and her husband stand up... and then a toddler, and another older couple. So much for less stress. *Here we go,* I think to myself. This couple has been waiting here for almost 40 minutes and they brought a child and extended family members. What a treat.

I still do not know why people bring anyone but their spouse to appointments, or even their spouses at times for that matter. Okay, I get the childcare thing, but if you are both here then can't the partner take the kid while I do your medical exam? And, in this case can't the mother-in-law take the kid while the couple enjoys some one-on-one time with the new addition? I will never know. But, the reality is this: I am going to have to simultaneously do my job, make sure a toddler isn't sticking things in outlets, overly apologize for being so late, and explain every little white spec on the screen to the mother-in-law who has never seen an ultrasound in her life. I can already feel the sweat under my armpits.

I want to express the fact that I love kids, they are the sweetest souls and if I was a teacher I would love to have them in my room exploring their environment. However, I am not a teacher. I am a sonographer. This is a medical examination and not a child proof room. I cannot watch your kid while also doing my extremely important job. So, if they are slamming on my keyboard, screaming inconsolably, or sticking paper clips in outlets, I am respectfully going to have to ask you to reschedule your appointment. As much as I wish I had eyes in the back of my head and twelve arms, I do not. I fully understand the constraints of childcare and other limitations but I also can't do my job properly given the latter. I also have constraints. Now, newborns who literally sleep in the carseat the entire time or teenagers who only look up from their phones when I yell FIRE, well maybe not then either, are the only two exceptions. You wouldn't take your toddler to your dental or pap smear appointments, would you? No, okay great now that we've cleared that up.

"Monica, can you please sit with Isabelle while the exam is being performed?" I hear Tanya direct her voice towards her mother-in-law as we enter the ultrasound room.

Thank God, a patient who gets it, I think to myself. I gesture to her husband to sit in the chair provided next to Tanya. Everyone surprisingly seems quite settled, given the fact that I wrongly assumed this may turn into a family reunion nightmare. Happily surprised I begin my speech.

"During the exam I am going to be assessing the baby, taking measurements, and checking the position. At the end of the exam we will find out an estimated weight of the baby and if there is cooperation, maybe get some photos." I always like to give the expectation that photos are only an option, given the fact that I cannot go inside of Tanya and turn the baby into the correct position for a perfect image. Although, most days I wish I could.

Everyone seems to nod silently in agreement, except Isabelle, the toddler; she is whining about some snack she doesn't have. So, as you can see even with the most well behaved humans in my room, it is still chaotic. There are still extra people I must address and extra noise that can be cause for distraction, but, overall, things are settled in our room for now, unless the building decides to set off an unplanned fire alarm, don't even get me started on the chaos of that. It may as well be a true fire with the way people run around like chickens with their heads cut off.

Tanya looks tired sitting on the ultrasound table. I am sure her brain is working just as hard as mine is to navigate and direct all the moving parts of her life right now. The difference is, hers never leaves but mine will walk out the door in about 60 minutes. She swings her legs up onto the footrest and lifts her shirt up, ready to tuck in any linens that I hand her.

"You must have done this before, you are a pro," I manage to get out soft enough for her ears and attention only.

She looks at me and just scoffs. Yep, she is exhausted. Her ankles look swollen, her hair is in a messy bun and I am almost certain that if she came to this appointment alone, she would fall asleep during the exam. This is surprisingly not uncommon, at least for women who are here just for routine scans.

I squeeze some of the warm ultrasound gel onto her belly and start my exam. The transducer camera is all tangled up and I step back for a moment to undo it. You would think I am doing ballerina tricks in here with the way these wires get all turned and twisted, but I literally go to the same exact position for every patient. I know, I know, not so ergonomically correct.

Tanya's husband is more interested in asking me questions about how I can type with my left hand than he is about the ultrasound images of his next child.

"Wow, you must be ambidextrous or something, how do you do that so fast with your left hand? Do people that are right handed have a harder time learning ultrasound?" He trails off asking question after question.

I step back into my designated spot at the machine and continue to assess the fetus. My only reply is a small chuckle. I guess I am also exhausted. Phew, I think to myself, only two more patients after this and I can go home. While I am in my own world, I hear a crash behind me. I shut my eyes and take a deep annoyed breath. As I glance behind me briefly I see my computer keyboard on the floor and the toddler standing there without an ounce of remorse. There are five adults in this room, two of them are occupied, can one of the other three please watch this child for the love of God.

"Let's not touch that anymore please Isabelle," I get out while looking back at my ultrasound screen, trying to do my job. I guess we can add babysitting to my scope of practice. I cannot safely have an unoccupied child in my room. I stop the exam and look around the room at all the adults.

"I cannot do my job unless someone is watching Isabelle. It is not a child proof room. Can someone please watch her so that I can finish my exam and get you all on your way?" I state in a very kind but direct manner.

"Otherwise we will need to reschedule for a time when you can come without your child." I repeat.

Once this information is understood I continue with the ultrasound. "It looks like your baby is head down, which is great, she doesn't want to look at us today, but that's okay." I mutter along as I move my hand up and down her abdomen, taking picture after picture for the doctors to review.

This is another part of ultrasound that no one seems to understand or talk about. Not even in school, at least not to this extent. When assessing your fetus, a sonographer must visualize multiple live portions of the exam. We are looking for different movements such as tone and gross body wiggles, practice breathing, and not only the heart rate but the rhythm as well. A still image can only give so much information. The doctors are not looking at a live video of each patient, they are looking at still images. It is my job to make sure these acts are present and within normal limits.

Like I have said before, if I don't see it or document it then the doctor can not tell you about it. I am the first line in diagnosing a normal or abnormal ultrasound result. This is why the title granted on my graduation certificate is "diagnostic" medical sonographer. As much as everyone, including the doctors themselves, tell you that we are not diagnosing, that is exactly what we are doing, even if we are not allowed to write it in the reports. I take that back. We cannot sign the reports, but you best believe we do all of the leg work in writing them. Sure, the providers go to school for like 40 years to do all, know all, and get paid all, but in this particular instance it's lost on me what their role is, when all they have to do is sign on the dotted line.

Tanya seems distracted. Due to the fact that none of her family members can wrangle a small toddler for 15 minutes, I would be too. Distraction is good, at least for me right now. I am already behind on my schedule and if she demands 3D images I am not going to get home tonight until 6:30 p.m.

She seems to ignore my mention of not being able to see the face of the baby today and that brings pure relief to my muscles, especially my sore shoulder. That means this exam is pretty much complete. Everything looks within normal limits, I have documented all my measurements, and I would say she would be all set to be on her way, until she sits up and asks, "So how much does the baby weigh?"

I am just barely finishing and telling her she can wipe up the gel on her stomach. I place the probe down and answer, "Let me get to my computer and I can tell you, give me just one minute."

Of course what I really mean is give a minute to get my keyboard off the ground and make sure my computer is still functioning and then I can give you the answer. Thankfully no damage was done other than logging me out of all twelve of my operating systems. Okay fine, three systems but still it feels like more most days.

Between the logging in and the slight malfunction of the communication between my ultrasound machine and the computer we have now been sitting here for ten extra minutes. That does not bode well for an annoyed pregnant mama, an antsy toddler, and three other extremely aloof adults. Finally everything miraculously starts to work.

"Your baby is weighing about 6 pounds, give or take, today," I say as I click through a couple of boxes on the screen.

Of course, we are never 100% accurate, we can get pretty close, but without the baby physically on the scale, this is just a best estimate. The next question, like clockwork, I can feel it coming.

"How long is the baby right now?" Tanya asks in conversation.

"We cannot determine that any more due to the fact that the baby is all curled up in there, it would be inaccurate, but they will measure once she is born," I reply as if I have said this a million times, because I have, in fact, said it a million times.

It seems that I have been able to get through this exam relatively easily. Everything is within normal limits and aside from the toddler situation, the actual child, not the absent minded adults, the overall experience was a breeze compared to the beginning of my day.

Tanya thanks me and herds her family with a swipe of her hands out the door. Tanya needs a nap which I hope she can get sooner than later. I wait until I assume there are more than an ears distance away and let out a huge sigh.

"Phew," I actually say out loud.

I slump down onto the computer chair and put my hands on my abdomen. My eyes start to close, but not long before my brain remembers that I still have another patient waiting. I probably have two waiting at this point, but thankfully I can now say that will be the last. Two more patients and my day is over and I can actually close my eyes and keep them shut for more than a millisecond.

4:03 p.m.

SOMEHOW I managed to get consistently 33 minutes behind from the moment I came back from my non-existent lunch break. My 3:30 p.m. patient has been in the waiting room for longer than I anticipated. It feels like I am running a 5k, my breath is actively faster than normal and my heart rate feels like it is through the roof. This can't be healthy. I have not even had a chance to sip my water this afternoon. I look at the sad three fourths full bottle on my desk and immediately feel my chapped lips and sense the looming headache I will surely have on my drive home. This makes me angry, which in turn does not make anything better. I protest and take a sip of water that turns into a five minute long chugging session. I deserve it. My brain analyzes that last thought, "I deserve it." I roll my eyes again, like I don't deserve to drink water at work. Now I know this isn't healthy or most likely legal, right? How did we get here? To this place of treating employees like they are numbers and patients like they are merely just appointments that fit into neatly organized time slots. Everything is dictated by insurance and drug companies. Providers are barely able to practice medicine in their own individualized capacity. But, that is a whole other conversation and topic for another day.

The clock reads 4:01 p.m. and by the time I get to the waiting room it's going to be a few minutes later. My heart rate spikes again as I come back to reality and orient myself to my next patient's chart.

Holly is here for a baseline follicle ultrasound. Remember those internal vaginal ultrasounds I was talking about at the beginning of my day? Yeah, one of those.

As I am briefly scanning through her chart, I realize this is not Holly's first rodeo with the internal wand. Holly is an infertility patient. She has been trying to get pregnant now for six years. She has had multiple losses resulting from early miscarriage to genetic complications further along in gestation. My eyes continue to read down line after line. She has done seven rounds of in vitro fertilization (IVF) so far and is planning on starting her eighth next month. I casually sit back and just cannot even imagine the stress, time, money, and emotional journey this woman has taken on.

At this clinic, we rarely see infertility patients. They are usually seen at a specific clinic solely to meet the needs of these patients. I probably see a handful per month on our schedule that are here for some sort of fertility ultrasound. That is nothing compared to the hundreds of patients we see per day.

Having a designated practice that addresses similar, extremely sensitive patient needs is way more desirable for a lot of reasons, hence why our clinic works directly with the infertility center down the road. I am familiar with the infertility world. This is one of the ultrasound rooms that we staff daily at one of our off site locations. I rotate there once or twice a week, but rarely do the patients get seen here at the outpatient OB/GYN office.

Holly's extensive history with IVF makes me curious about her journey and the strength it takes to continue even through presumed failure. Reading through her chart I ironically feel a small burst of energy once again. It's almost like her strength and determination seeps into me from just the mere thought of her story. Maybe it is that or the half gallon of water that I just chugged, but either way.

I set my room up for the internal ultrasound with a sheet, the stirrups, and the cold gel that literally feels like it is from the arctic. That's what you get with things that are sterile, they will never be warm. At least I know that I won't have to explain what a vaginal ultrasound is to this woman. She could probably perform her own at this point with the dozens she has had in the past.

My muscle memory kicks in and I head out the door of my room, down the hall, and back to the waiting room for hopefully one of my last journeys today. I could probably walk these halls in my sleep, upside down, and with my eyes closed at this point.

When I open the waiting room door the room is about half full. You never notice just how many pregnant women are in one room until you are calling in the only non-pregnant woman to her appointment.

"Holly," I call out into the room.

My back to the door, my foot props it open and my eyes scan the room while I wait for a response.

"Holly?" I call again after no one seems to be answering my summons.

Finally, a young woman looks over at me as she is taking out one of her earbuds,

"Did you say Holly?" she questioned.

"I am so sorry." She is now frantically collecting her things and apologizing.

It is me who should really be the one to apologize as I am

not retrieving her for her appointment until about 30 minutes after the scheduled time.

"No need to rush, would you like to use the bathroom before the exam?" I motion to the bathroom door as we make our way back down the hallway.

Holly declines, as she continues to shove all of her belongings into her large tote bag.

Sitting in a waiting room full of visibly pregnant women must be such a mentally difficult thing to endure when that is literally the one thing you are working so hard towards, such as in Holly's case. You can see why most of these women would rather go to a specialized fertility clinic, as to surround themselves with other people going through a similar journey, rather than sitting in a room full of achieved dreams. It is tough enough to go through IVF, never mind throwing all of the other things life has in store for us into the mix.

On the other hand, it could provide hope to Holly who can possibly envision her future goals. Either way, Holly is here, she wants to be here, she is working hard to be here and I really hope I can give her some good news today instead of the latter.

I barely get the door shut before Holly throws her bag down on the chair and starts to get undressed. She knows the drill, one too many of these and you will also want to get them over and done with. I get it. I pretend to be working on my computer to give her the privacy she deserves, but it seems she does not want any. She makes it over to the exam table with the sheet half covering her lap and one of her earbuds still in.

She lets out an audible breath and asks, "Will these results get to my provider today?"

I can tell she is so annoyed with this process and just simply wants to achieve the end result sooner than later, I mean who wouldn't? Patients going through IVF have the most turbulent emotions that I have ever witnessed. One day they get good numbers and they are over the moon and the next tragedy strikes and they are back into a deep dark hole of despair and anger. This makes me prepared for basically anything because wouldn't you also be a hot mess if this was your constant battle?

The bravery, utter guts, and courage it takes just to start the IVF process is an incredible physiologic feat in and of itself, nevermind all the details and deadlines that come with the journey. It is almost like going through the stages of grief over and over again until finally, hopefully, by the grace of a miracle and a little science, you get to bring home your bundle of joy.

"Yes, I will fax them over as soon as we are done here," I quickly reply to Holly as if this is going to make a difference at 4:00 p.m. on a weekday. These women depend on same day results. I have no idea how this is going to happen this late in the day, but unfortunately or frankly fortunately, this is out of my circle of control. I am going to do my part, fax the results, and hope the best for her. Holly is completely checked out, she is laid back on the table, feet in the stirrups, scrolling through her phone without the slightest bit of eye contact. I check to see if she made it far enough to the edge of the table, but Holly could even scoot back a bit and still be in the perfect position. She gets the overachiever award in scooting, not that she desired to attain that whatsoever.

A lot of women who go through IVF do not end up with a child. All that money, effort, shots, ultrasounds, and bloodwork and not much to show for it other than some bruises and an empty bank account. I have asked countless women about their journeys and I have traveled beside these women, metaphorically holding their hands and cheering them on from the sidelines. Making the first decision to start this process has to be grueling, knowing that the outcome is not guaranteed. But, on the other hand it must also be exciting and hopeful to know that there is this part of science that could, in many cases, help them achieve their family dreams. My mind tries to wrap around the world these IVF patients encounter, but without personal experience this perspective will never be possible.

I lift the sheet that is covering Holly's lap slightly and begin to hand her the ultrasound probe.

"I am just going to hand you this for you to guide," I start to say, hoping she is listening to me.

She quickly grabs the probe and nearly flawlessly inserts the camera. She immediately goes back to scrolling on her phone. I can take a hint and so I stay mostly silent during the exam, assuming she would just like to get this over with and get on with her day. Again, completely understandable. Usually I talk about the weather or the coming weekend versus last weekend. Although, if a scan falls on a Wednesday I never really know what to ask the patient about. I can't really ask if they had a good weekend prior nor can I refer to any future weekend plans. Wednesdays really put a cramp in my patient small talk experience, maybe that's my cue to take Wednesdays off. Thankfully Holly doesn't appear to be in a small talk kind of mood; my lucky day.

As I am lost in thought about taking time off, Holly asks, "What is my largest follicle measuring?"

I have to bring myself back to reality for a minute, at this point my learned memory takes over when I am not prompted to talk during scans.

"Let me just finish up with the uterus and I will let you

know," I reply hesitating a bit.

Even though giving Holly a single number is not going to tell her anything one way or the other it still feels like I am the one responsible for the fate of this round of IVF. It's as if when I don't find a large enough or small enough follicle it's on me, all my fault somehow. Obviously this is not the case, but it doesn't make it feel any better. I want to give these patients good news every single time, which is the same as all my patients.

"The largest follicle is measuring 16 millimeters," I tell Holly as I am taking out the ultrasound probe.

To be honest this measurement could go either way for her treatment. I do not know her specific plan or bloodwork results so I have no way of knowing. I will let her doctor discuss all of this with her. Holly however has other plans.

"Okay, so does that mean I am ready for the trigger shot?" She asks as if I am the knower of all information.

"I am not sure, that is going to have to be something that you discuss with your doctor," I reply.

I can tell she is slightly annoyed but also understanding that this isn't the time or place for that question. I get it, it's so hard to wait for an answer that you do want and honestly probably even harder to wait for one that you don't. I express my understanding to Holly as she is getting dressed, again without any care of my presence in the room. I turn towards my computer and finish the report, in hopes to get this faxed out in time for her doctor's office to review the results.

Holly is now dressed and completely paying attention, no earbuds, no scrolling; she is looking me straight in the eyes.

She starts to walk towards the exit door and says, "Thank you for your time, have a great night."

It's moments like these that remind me that the work I am doing matters. I can feel the gratitude pouring out of her like a waterfall. It means something much bigger than me.

"You're welcome," I say looking directly back at her, hoping she knows how much I wish for her journey to end exactly the way she hopes it will.

4:16 p.m.

I CAN'T believe that I am about to take in my last patient of the day, albeit 15 minutes late, but hey not that shabby. I should be wrapping up my reports, cleaning my room, and stocking shelves for the next day at this time of night. My shift ends at 4:30 p.m. and I am an hourly employee; I would like to leave at my scheduled time. Overtime and me are not friends anymore. More days than not I do not leave on time. I guess I could technically talk to my boss about this, but what would that do? Either the patients would suffer or my coworkers would suffer, so I suck it up and head to the waiting room for the last time today.

Lauren is here for an exam because her fetus is measuring small, or "size less than dates." This basically means that at one of her prenatal appointments the doctor measured her belly and the size did not match how far along she is in her pregnancy. I am once again hoping, very strongly, that this is just a fluke measurement and this baby is completely normal. However my instincts are driving me towards the opposite direction once I see Lauren stand up in the waiting room.

After calling her name out into the now empty room, Lauren stands up easily and starts walking towards me. She is supposed to be 37 weeks along, only three weeks away from delivery. Instead, she looks like she is about 20 weeks and to be honest, barely pregnant at all. She is tiny. This does not always mean much. I have seen super tall women who can easily hide their pregnancy the whole time, yet the growth of the baby is normal throughout. But Lauren is not that tall and I have a sinking feeling this exam is going to take much longer than I originally intended.

Lauren glides past me as I hold the door open for her. Without hesitation she turns her head back in my direction and asks, "Is this going to take long, because I need to pick my son up from daycare before 5:30 p.m.?"

Clearly she is a little miffed that I am taking her in for her appointment late. I get it, truly I do, I also would like to be on my way out the door but alas here we are. The other caveat to this situation is if things are not normal with her scan, she is going to be here much longer than she intended.

"As long as the baby cooperates and everything looks good it shouldn't take too long," I say, as I do to almost every patient who asks this *exact same question.*

It really all depends on the baby. Are they active and alert or are they asleep and lazy? Is the growth normal or abnormal? There are way too many factors at play for me to give a black and white answer to this question. Thankfully I have a pretty good scripted response in my head for it.

We make it down the hallway and into my ultrasound room. Lauren walks in and sets down her things on the chair beside the exam table.

"I am just going to go to the bathroom really quick before we start," she says as she scurries out the door.

I purposefully left out that question due to the fact that I know we are late and she is on a time schedule but by all means delay the inevitable a little longer. I start to pick up and clean what I can while she is out of the room, preparing my things secretly to rush out the door once this is over.

When I say rush I literally mean rush, like running out the door without looking back.

Not surprisingly it takes Lauren about one minute to use the restroom and return. She is efficient. Once back in the room she sits down comfortably on the exam table and prepares for the ultrasound. I use the remote control for the table to lift her lower legs into a neutral position while reclining the back of the chair. Tucking the towel into her lower pants she lies back.

"If you could just scoot closer to me that would be helpful," I ask hoping she will oblige.

She does and we are ready to start the ultrasound and figure out the fate of our afternoon together.

My shoulder is on its last leg, I can feel the pins and needles in my finger tips and the pain scoring down my right scapula. My stomach cannot live off of any more ibuprofen but that's the going cure for my work related pain and injuries. *Major* eye roll, like my eyes hurt with this one. I cannot express enough how ignorant the employee healthcare system truly is.

It is the system versus the people, and how needed the people who run the system are and how broken the system that employs them really is. My internal anger starts to burn and I can feel my heart beat faster and faster.

Someone in the field of ultrasound/work related injury/ employee wellness needs to listen and take notes again. Recall that about 90 percent of sonographers scan in pain. Not nine percent; *ninety*. That is basically everyone unless you are brand new out of school and haven't had time to injure yourself yet. Hospitals do very little to educate and support our constant ergonomic needs.

I hope that someday, in the very near future, employee health systems recognize the dire need for programs that not only treat but prevent workplace injuries. I know that ultrasound can't be the only career that is super high on the list of injuries sustained in hospitals. I see nurses lifting patients that are over 300 pounds and janitorial staff constantly reaching or bending in awkward ways. We can come together to make this better. A healthy and pain free medical employee means happy and healthier patients, right? Yes, 100% I will stick by this philosophy all day every day. It seems the healthcare system really just sees it as, *well if you can't handle it you can leave and we will hire someone else to do the job, probably for cheaper.* There is no value in employees anymore, unless you're a physician. I realize this rant in my head needs to end and I need to concentrate on the patient in front of me. I take a long deep breath and focus my eyes on the screen.

My right hand is scanning Lauren's belly with my camera, up and down looking for any signs of disease. I am checking on the baby and the uterus very carefully. My left hand is running the ultrasound machine knobs and toggle switches. My brain is navigating between my physical hands moving and my eyes assessing the image on the screen. Pretty wild when you think about it. I would say a very ambidextrous job. Kudos to the husband earlier for acknowledging this fact.

The image starts to wiggle up and down with the baby's movements. Good this little one is already acing the test, I think to myself.

"Baby is moving great in there," I assure Lauren.

I can feel the anxious energy coming from her, for both the wellbeing of her unborn baby and the deadline of her other child's daycare pick up. Lauren gives a slight smile, but her eyes remain locked on the patient viewing monitor.

"Do you know if it's a boy or a girl?" I ask.

"It's another boy, houseful of boys," she replies.

The amniotic fluid around the baby measures normal, the placenta looks great except for a couple cystic areas, and the baby passes the biophysical profile with flying colors. He even practiced his breathing for the entire exam. This is basically an exercise that fetuses do to train the diaphragm to be ready when they are born to do actual breathing.

Now it is time to measure the baby, the real reason Lauren was sent here today. Lauren is getting antsy. My arm is burning now in pain but I have to muster the strength to carry on for ten more minutes.

I freeze the ultrasound image on the screen and begin measuring the baby's head. These measurements are assisted by technology and different mathematical algorithms; thankfully because that was not always the case. Once I get all the measurements my machine sends the information over to my computer and shoots out a percentile and estimated weight.

"What is the baby weighing?" Lauren asks when she sees the measurements on the screen.

"I need to get a measurement of his belly and leg bone and then we will review everything," I reply while glancing over at her.

I know she just wants to hurry up and get out of here.

"My last son was an average birth weight so I am sure this one will be just fine," she reasons.

"Every baby is so different," I reply because my eyes can already see the smaller than expected measurements of the baby's head.

It is measuring about five weeks behind, which is not great, but not too worrisome since he is passing the rest of the exam. I make my way to the abdomen and leg of the baby and document those measurements. All seem to be lagging about five weeks behind from her gestational age. Because of how far along she is I know that the doctor will most likely make the recommendation for her to go straight to labor and delivery for more monitoring and possible early delivery. Oh what a way to end the day.

I let this sink in before immediately dropping the news on Lauren. She is going to be in shock and I am going to be here for another twenty minutes, *minimum*, between finding a doctor and calling Labor and Delivery to give them a heads up.

"I got everything I need, you can sit up, wipe off the gel and I will get you the measurements in just a minute," I promise her.

I click some buttons on my ultrasound machine and place the transducer back in its slot for the last time today. Good riddance. I feel like chucking it out the window, but that would be a costly attempt at revenge.

"I do have a concern with the growth of your baby," I say to Lauren. I am sitting across from her looking directly into her annoyed eyes.

"Okay, so what does that mean?" She snaps back.

"I am going to go get the doctor to discuss all of it with you, I will be right back," I quickly reply, half way out the door, leaving her no time for a response.

I shuffle down the quiet hallway, crossing my fingers that the doctor has not yet left. He is not supposed to leave until the last ultrasound patient is finished, however that is not always the case. And I only say "He" here because there is only one of them that disobeys this rule and he happens to be the one here this afternoon. I can see from the corner that the lights are off in his office. My body sinks, but then I peek my head in and there he is in the flesh, thank the good Lord.

"Hi, Cassie, what do you have for me?" He says almost

immediately as I walk in.

What is he, a mind reader in his spare time? I fumble my words, but get them out clear enough. Without responding to me he picks up the phone and dials Labor and Delivery.

"Yeah, hi is this the attending? I have a 37 weeker that will be coming over shortly for monitoring and possible delivery," he barks into the phone as if the person on the other line is hard of hearing. Great, well at least that's one less phone call that I have to make before I leave. He puts the phone back on the receiver and jets past me out the door as if I am a ghost.

"I am in room three," I shout down the hall as I run to catch up with him.

I can tell he is equally annoyed to have to deal with this situation at quitting time, but what can we do? It is what it is and we can't predict the outcomes of our four o'clock patients. For some reason they usually end up being the most complicated cases of the day. Maybe that's Murphy's Law or pure coincidence but either way I'm not into it and clearly neither is the doctor.

We quickly reach my ultrasound room and he opens the door while knocking. I follow silently behind him. Lauren is sitting in the chair on the opposite side of the room, waiting not so patiently for some answers. She perks up slightly when he walks through the door and her eyes look red. I am sure she is completely stressed out; this is not what she was expecting at all. But, that's pregnancy, expect the unexpected. I feel cynical saying this, but after seeing thousands of pregnant women I think I have earned the right.

The doctor grabs the chair on wheels and sits down across from Lauren.

"My name is Dr. Ward. Nice to meet you Lauren. So, it looks like today your baby is measuring less than expected by ultrasound. He is measuring about five weeks behind, which puts him at less than the first percentile for growth. This is slightly concerning and my recommendation would be to admit you to the hospital for some extra monitoring and possibly an early delivery of this baby."

As soon as he finishes his small speech I look over at the patient and she looks like a deer caught in headlights. The doctor continues, "At this point the baby would grow better on the outside rather than on the inside of your uterus which is why we recommend you head over to Labor and Delivery following our discussion."

Lauren looks at me to confirm his words, but I just nod and look at the doctor. Patients do this a lot, like I am some keeper of the answers they actually want to hear and not the ones the doctor has. I think especially when they are here alone they just need some comfort, someone other than the doctor to say *hey, this sucks and I am here to listen.* Subconsciously they have written off the doctor as evil for a moment and me as someone who can shine any hope on the situation.

"So I have to go over there like right now? I need to pick up my son." Lauren replies.

"I would call someone to help with that if possible, maybe your partner or a relative. It is my recommendation that you go directly to the hospital," The doctor states once again.

Again we cannot force people to follow our recommendations but we can strongly encourage, which is clearly what he is doing. Lauren and Dr. Ward go back and forth for a few minutes regarding specific questions that she has when finally he leaves and trails back down the hallway to his office. I feel the need to reassure Lauren again that everything is okay, it's just best to be cautious. She agrees and starts furiously texting and dialing numbers into her cell phone. I show her out the back door.

"Good luck to you," I call as she turns the corner to hopefully proceed to the hospital, but time will only tell.

"Thanks," she chimes back down the hall while holding the phone to her ear and rummaging through her bag simultaneously.

At this point just about everyone else has left for the day and the hallways are eerily quiet. I step back into my room and finish up my end of day duties before turning off my ultrasound machine. Hearing the machine power down immediately brings my blood pressure back to normal. Once that shuts down the entire room is silent. I don't like it at all, so I make haste and power walk to clock out for the day.

5:02 p.m.

TWO MINUTES past five, 32 minutes past the end of my shift. Some days it's 28 minutes, others it's one, but rarely it's on time. Never is it early. As soon as my badge beeps on the machine to clock out my entire body relaxes. I did it, I am free. It sounds like I am exiting prison or something, not that they are similar, but the feeling of being trapped and unable to leave is at the top of my mind some days. Today being one of them.

Stepping out into the fresh air my lungs catch and I open my eyes towards the horizon, taking in the sunset that is left. Before hopping into my car to drive home I slowly breathe in this moment. A moment of serenity. My car beeps to signal unlocking and I get into the driver's seat. I take my badge off from around my neck and place it back into the depths of my never ending bag. My shoulder aches and my brain hurts. I briefly recall my day, trying to process all that was consumed. Then I think, better not. Throwing those thoughts and emotions into a hidden compartment within my brain, I put my seat belt on and the car in drive, knowing full well I will be back to do it all over again tomorrow.

EPILOGUE

FAST FORWARD a few years and a pandemic later. Two years of working non stop through the pandemic following the birth of my daughter, Eleanor, in October 2019 has felt like a time warp. It either feels like time is flying or standing still. Maybe that is parenthood or maybe that's the unfortunate circumstances we found ourselves in during this unprecedented time.

It definitely hit me hard on both a mental health and personal level. The possible tragedies and miracles that come with childbirth almost flawlessly mirror the realities of the current world. As almost everyone can say, I am exhausted. I have since taken a step back from my full time hours in maternal fetal medicine and transitioned to a part time career at an infertility clinic. This gives me more time for my family, which is what I truly desired. I do hope to return to a more capable full time aspect one day, but for now my personal health and family need to come first.

When I finally made the decision to leave, I had also been looking at masked, emotionless faces for years. Patients also looked at the blue covering on my nonexistent face, searching for answers that would not be found. We were both able to hide in a way that did not benefit these delicate situations. I literally had to relearn how to manage my facial muscles post mask wearing. Things changed. I was more distant from my patients, for better or worse I don't know, but I did know that it was time for me to move on.

Less truly is more; stepping back from the hospital chaos has taught me that invaluable lesson time and time again. I put my career and my patients first for almost ten years. I think that's the sin and the beauty of providing healthcare, it means exceptional care at the cost of possibly losing ourselves in the journey along the way. Like I have said before and I will say it again, I have no idea how some people manage to navigate a hospital based career for thirty, forty plus years. Kudos and Godspeed. You are keeping the healthcare system afloat, well you and all the clueless but eager new grads and residents.

As much as I emphasize the traumatic events that happen within the walls of the high risk clinic, there are so many of the happy and exciting ones that happen just as often if not more.

Not everything inside that building is heartache. Some days it feels like it, but there are a high percentage of pregnancies that turn out relatively normal. The hard cases leave a larger mark in some ways than all the good and positive situations. I think that is simply due to the fact that we are dealing with life and death, not merely a break up or job loss.

I wanted to bring a sense of understanding and community to the complexities of pregnancy. Even if your pregnancy went completely smooth and couldn't have been easier, it is anything but that for someone else.

There are multiple other stories that I omitted. Stories of third trimester losses and extended hospital stays without a delivery in sight. Patients who have carried a pregnancy until the day before delivery and when I put my camera down on the belly for one more ultrasound, there is no heartbeat. Immediate grief taken on by myself, even for mere seconds before I had to give that gut wrenching news. Patients who are my friends that I get to deliver amazing and exciting news to. Patients who have been trying to conceive for years and finally get to see the heartbeat of their embryo. My nearly eleven year career is filled with more grief than I can stand to discuss, but it is also filled with lots and lots of joy.

Since I initially wrote this book, I have experienced multiple miscarriages. I can share in the feelings of loneliness, anger, and confusion. When the story does not end the way I envisioned it. I am endlessly grateful for my daughter.

No experience is too minor to feel. I would do anything to own a magic wand and take away all the heartache and unexpected challenges. Without any magic powers I try my best every day to show up and be there for my patients through all of it; the good, the bad, and the unimaginable.

We are all put together by the microscopic cells that create us. Not one of those cells can be out of place or things can go awry, and that's my job, to assess the detours and deficiencies. The ups and the downs. The peaks and the valleys. The lovely and devastating waves through pregnancy.

ACKNOWLEDGEMENTS

THIS STORY could not have been written without the unwavering support of my husband, Neal Jandreau. His continued encouragement to persevere through all of my roadblocks is unmatched. For years he has helped me to follow my dream of making this book a reality and has also been an incredible guide. He organized my thoughts when I was lost, gave me a shoulder to cry on when I was sad and has celebrated every step of the way alongside me. For a decade he gave me a solid foundation for my extreme stress and exhaustion to land, day after day, shift after shift. His insurmountable knowledge about all the details of publishing, book layout and design, and helping my vision of the cover art come to life has been remarkable. This book would not exist without him.

My daughter, Eleanor, is young, but I want to recognize and

196 | Waves: A Day in the Life of a Sonographer

thank her for even her unconscious ability to bear with me during new motherhood, a pandemic, and a completely and utterly chaotic career.

Deep gratitude to my close family, friends, and coworkers for taking this trip alongside me. Thank you for always answering my texts and calls when I was overthinking everything and for continuing to be excited about the end goal.

I want to thank a dear friend, Brittany Winslow, for constantly challenging me and asking the tough questions. She was able to dissect exactly what I wanted to say and bring clarity to my work. She has been a tremendous mentor throughout this process.

I want to thank Josh Pahigian for giving me invaluable insights into the world of editing and writing. I know my grammar can sometimes be quite the hurdle. Thank you for your time.

A huge thank you to Danielle Brown, who is the Director of Diagnostic Medical Sonography at the Maine College of Health Professions. She has been a colleague of mine for many, many years and has experienced most of these stories both in tandem with me and in her current role in education.

I want to thank all the Doctors I have worked with for their incredible fortitude and patience. Without the rigorous training from the physicians over the years I would not have half the knowledge that I have today.

I want to sincerely recognize all of my fellow sonographers in all specialties, from the ambitious new graduates to the seasoned veterans. The work you do is beyond important and changes lives every day, both expected and unexpected. The emotional, physical, and mental strength it takes to work with patients of unborn fetuses is truly extraordinary.

Finally, I want to thank all of the patients I have scanned and had the pleasure of meeting over the years for inspiring me to create something that can be shared with the world.

ABOUT THE AUTHOR

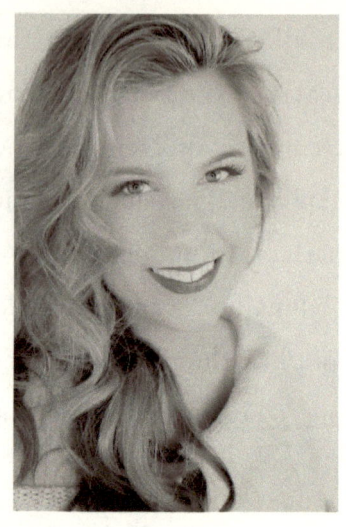

Cassandra McGinnity (Cassie) is a seasoned sonographer who has dedicated her career to specializing in Women's Health. She graduated from The University of Southern Maine with a B.S. in Health Sciences. From there she pursued ultrasound and graduated in 2014 from the New Hampshire Technical Institute as a Diagnostic Medical Sonographer. She holds four ARDMS board credentials including Abdomen/Small Parts, Obstetrics/Gynecology, and Fetal Echocardiography. She served as an adjunct professor of the OB/GYN ultrasound course at NHTI in 2017/2018. She is a member of the Maine Sonographers Association and has participated in multiple medical conferences representing ultrasound. Cassie loves being a mom and spending time with her family. She enjoys hiking, photography, reading, traveling, and exploring the outdoors in her home state of Maine.

www.ingramcontent.com/pod-product-compliance
Lightning Source LLC
Chambersburg PA
CBHW031514120626
46545CB00005B/1873